WHEN
SOMEONE
YOU LOVE HAS
A MENTAL
ILLNESS

WHEN SOMEONE YOU LOVE HAS A MENTAL ILLNESS

A Handbook for Family, Friends, and Caregivers

REBECCA WOOLIS, M.F.T.

Foreword by Agnes B. Hatfield, Ph.D.

Jeremy P. Tarcher/Penguin
a member of
Penguin Group (USA) Inc.
New York

Most Tarcher/Penguin books are available at special quantity discounts for bulk purchase for sales promotions, premiums, fund-raising, and educational needs. Special books or book excerpts also can be created to fit specific needs.

For details, write Penguin Group (USA) Inc. Special Markets, 375 Hudson Street, New York, NY 10014.

PUBLISHER'S NOTE

Every effort has been made to ensure that the information contained in this book is complete and accurate. However, neither the publisher nor the author is engaged in rendering professional advice or services to the individual reader. The ideas, procedures, and suggestions contained in this book are not intended as a substitute for consulting with your physician. All matters regarding your health require medical supervision. Neither the author nor the publisher shall be liable or responsible for any loss or damage allegedly arising from any information or suggestion in this book.

While the author has made every effort to provide accurate telephone numbers and Internet addresses at the time of publication, neither the publisher nor the author assumes any responsibility for errors, or for changes that occur after publication.

The author welcomes your comments and questions.
Please write to:
Rebecca Woolis
925 The Almeda
Berkeley, CA 94707

Jeremy P. Tarcher/Penguin
a member of
Penguin Group (USA) Inc.
375 Hudson Street
New York, NY 10014
www.penguin.com

Copyright © 1992, 2003 by Rebecca Woolis, M.F.T.
All rights reserved. This book, or parts thereof, may not be reproduced in any form without permission. Published simultaneously in Canada

Library of Congress Cataloging-in-Publication Data

Woolis, Rebecca.
    When someone you love has a mental illness : a handbook for family, friends, and caregivers / Rebecca Woolis ; foreword by Agnes B. Hatfield.—
[Rev. & expanded ed.]
        p.   cm.
    Includes bibliographical references and index.
    ISBN 0-87477-695-3 (pbk. : alk. paper)
    1. Mentally ill—Home care.   2. Mentally ill—Care.   3. Mentally ill—Family relationships.   4. Mentally ill—Life skills guides.   I. Title.
RC439.5.W65   2003
362.2'4—dc21   2003055233

Design by Mauna Eichner

Printed in the United States of America

In loving memory of my mother,
Malvina Woolis,
and
in deep appreciation of my father,
Sol Woolis,
whose unfaltering encouragement and
confidence in me often exceeds my own.

The revised edition is dedicated to
Sarah Elizabeth Adams
and
Cameron Jeffrey Adams,
two delightful, bright young people
who add joy to my life
and help me stay in touch
with the younger generation
and "popular culture."

Contents

Quick Reference Guides

Acknowledgments

I HAVE MANY PEOPLE to thank for their contributions to the classes I taught and the educational support groups I led, all of which culminated in what I offer in this book. I am very grateful to Chris Amenson, Ph.D., for his generosity with the material he compiled for his classes, as well as his lecture notes, knowledge, and guidance when I began the Family Support Program. Much of that material is based on the work done by Paul Liberman, M.D., and the UCLA Clinical Research Center for Schizophrenia and Psychiatric Rehabilitation, which Dr. Liberman directs, along with the work of other pioneers in the field of family education: Ian Falloon, M.D.; Jeffrey Boyd, Ph.D.; Christine McGill, M.S.W.; E. Fuller Torrey, M.D.; Kayla Bernheim, Ph.D.; and Agnes Hatfield, Ph.D.—to name a few. Information in the revised edition has also been informed by the work of Xavier Amador, Ph.D., Mary Ellen Copeland, M.S., and Terence Gorski.

I appreciate the encouragement and support provided me by Buckelew Houses under the able guidance of Jay Zlotnick, executive director. He and the board of directors had the foresight to allow me to develop a program for families before it was a fashionable thing to do.

I thank Rex Dickens, who was most generous with his time and with the material he compiled for siblings and adult children of people with mental illness. He helped me keep their perspective in mind.

I am grateful to Jeanette Gurevitch for providing me with numerous needed nudges in order for me to pursue the notion of publishing my work. She will be missed by many.

I appreciate the help Peter Beren provided in organizing my embryonic material into a proposal ready to submit to a publisher.

I thank Aidan Kelly and Rick Benzel, who showed me what a wonderful job a professional editor can do with a manuscript.

I am deeply grateful to all the families I have worked with throughout the San Francisco Bay Area who have shared with me their lives and pain and taught me what I needed to teach and write for others. Stephanie Draper will always be remembered for her encouragement and tireless work on behalf of families and people struggling with mental illness.

In writing the additions to the 2003 edition, I thank Bonita Houses Inc., an excellent agency doing pioneering work in providing treatment and services to people with a dual diagnosis. It was during the four years I directed the residential treatment program there that I gained much valuable first-hand experience with and knowledge about such consumers struggling with a dual diagnosis and their families. I offer a special note of appreciation to Dr. Floyd Brown, Medical Director of Bonita Houses, one of the most knowledgeable and enjoyable psychiatrists with whom I have ever had the good fortune of working. He provided many hours of invaluable consultation about clients and the medication charts in this edition. I thank Rick Crispino, Executive Director, and Terry Rubin-Ortiz, LCSW Clinical Director, for their support, wisdom, and knowledge.

Jay Mahler's feedback and perspective about the consumer movement was extremely helpful. His firsthand experience and many years of dedicated work in the field have made a significant contribution to the well-being of many consumers. I thank Mary and Fritz Blume for reviewing early drafts and offering sound suggestions.

I thank my dear friends and relatives Jan Wiener, Ellie Waxman, William Woolis, and Evelyn Gross for their constant love, support, and encouragement in pursuing the revision of my original work. Additionally, I thank Jan Wiener for her valuable editorial help.

Foreword

A LITTLE MORE THAN two decades ago people began paying attention to the role that families play in the lives of their mentally ill relatives. Families found themselves in the tremendously difficult position of serving as primary caretakers of their seriously disturbed relatives although they had little or no understanding of their relatives' disorders or how to cope with them. The enormity of the burden that these families faced eventually came to light through a number of surveys and first-person accounts, which made it clear that if the movement toward community care was to survive, appropriate assistance would need to be given to caregiving relatives.

The social context in which these families were operating was changing: the traditional idea that families were etiological agents in their relatives' illnesses was fading due to lack of credible evidence; developments in biological psychiatry were rapidly changing our concept of what mental illnesses are; and the voices of the organized family movement were insisting on their right to define family needs.

Providers first responded to families by offering them the traditional individual and family therapies in which they were experienced. Studies showed that these therapies were not widely accepted by their clients. Families resisted being defined as patients in need of treatment or therapy. Their problem, they believed, was their need for an understanding of mental illnesses and their treatments, as well as a knowledge of resources in the community and of practical coping and management skills they could use at home. They were asking for education and training to prepare themselves for their new career as family caregivers.

What followed was nearly two decades of effort by a range of providers and educators to develop the most useful materials and the most efficacious approaches to teaching families the knowledge and skills they require. This book by Rebecca Woolis is a culmination of two decades of thinking about how best to help families.

Families who read this book will find their most urgent questions addressed in a manner that is sensitive, practical, and authoritative. They will encounter a thorough and accurate description of the major mental illnesses and the most respected current treatments, as well as useful suggestions for home management. Relatives will learn to deal with their own intense feelings and to solve problems more skillfully. In this book Rebecca Woolis talks to families with a gentle voice and an empathic understanding of what families are going through. The clarity of the information and the frequent Quick Reference Guides make this a welcome volume that is indeed user-friendly.

Agnes B. Hatfield, Ph.D.

Preface

THIS BOOK IS INTENDED as a handbook for families and friends of people who suffer from a mental illness. Whether the ill person is an adolescent or an adult, whether that person is living at home, in a hospital, in a sheltered environment, or on the streets, the entire family can benefit from learning to understand that person and how to best deal with him or her on a day-to-day basis.

For centuries, our culture has been struggling to understand the phenomenon known as mental illness. Artists, philosophers, theologians, and, more recently, psychiatrists and psychologists have given us a variety of images of people considered to be mad or insane. People suffering from a mental illness have experiences quite different from ours. They often cannot distinguish reality from their own fantasies. Their perceptions of the world are grossly distorted, and their moods may swing dramatically from one extreme to the other.

Sometimes people experience symptoms for brief periods. This may be a result of a life, spiritual, or identity crisis. In these cases, when the crisis is resolved, the condition passes. Symptoms may also occur as a reaction to a traumatic event or in response to taking a mind- or mood-altering drug. When, however, symptoms persist in a severe and disabling way for long periods, we now consider these symptoms to be caused by two groups of psychiatric conditions, *schizophrenia* and *major affective disorders*. These conditions are the most serious forms of mental illness.

Mental illnesses exist throughout the world, in every culture and country, regardless of custom, race, religion, economic condition, child-rearing practices, or political orientation. Different societies think about and treat their members with mental illness in very different ways. Some cultures consider them special or close to the gods, while others consider them bad, sick, or evil. It is this variable more than any other that determines the quality of life for people with mental illness and those who are close to them.

Our own culture presents a wide range of images of madness. Some views romanticize mental illness. Others hold that insanity is the only sane adaptation to an insane world, or that our society is insane and that our way of life drives people mad. While these beliefs may be partly true, they do not address the very real suffering experienced on a daily basis by people who have a mental illness, nor do they consider the heartache of their families and friends.

Worse than those who glorify mental illness are those who make pariahs of people with mental illness. Such a lack of understanding and compassion often exacerbates the symptoms of the illness, and perpetuates the suffering.

Our society lacks a clear and healthy approach to people with mental illness. The tragedy in this is that although we have the know-how to create environments in which people with mental illness can thrive to the fullest extent possible given the nature of the illnesses, our culture has never chosen to do so on a consistent long-term basis. Part of the problem is that we lack the financial commitment necessary to translate our store of knowledge, research, and experience into programs and services that are available to all who need them.

Many myths and misconceptions about people with mental illness run rampant in this country. Television, magazines, newspapers, and books have convinced the general public that all people with mental illness (they call them "the mentally ill") are psychotic killers or geniuses with split personalities. I find it sad and infuriating that people with mental illness are so misunderstood and misrepresented. Many of the people I have worked with who suffer from schizophrenia or major affective disorders are among the most gentle, endearing people I have ever known. They would like nothing more than to be able to be productive members of society who can think and act as most others do.

When Someone You Love Has a Mental Illness corrects the common misbeliefs about mental illness and presents in simple, everyday language the information needed to understand the world of people with mental illness and to be more comfortable with them. It provides relatives and friends with the tools necessary to deal with an array of behaviors and symptoms that are alien and frightening when you are unfamiliar with them. Ultimately, its goal is to help minimize the pain and suffering that these tragically disabling illnesses cause both the people afflicted with the illnesses and those who are close to them.

MY OWN JOURNEY

I was born in 1947 in the Bronx, New York. I completed my undergraduate work in psychology at the City College of New York in 1969. My first employment in the field of mental health also occurred in New York City, at Roosevelt Hospital's Child and Youth Project. The experience and training I received there from my supervisor-mentor Barbara Goodman Ph.D., a most knowledgeable, down-to-earth, and encouraging psychologist, made a lasting impression on me.

In 1970, I moved to California. I received a master's degree in clinical psychology from John F. Kennedy University in 1973. My first experience with people with major mental illness was during an internship in that program. I began working full-time with people with mental illness in 1976 and have continued doing so in some capacity ever since. I became a licensed Marriage and Family Therapist (M.F.T.) in 1978. I spent several years as a line staff in an intensive residential treatment program of Buckelew Houses. I was the Program Director for the following five years. In 1982, prompted by the glaring need I saw for families to have more contact with mental-health professionals, more support, and more information available to them, I began a Family Support Program for the agency. Since then, I have directed or been involved with various behavioral-health programs and services, including an adolescent substance-abuse unit, case-management services, a residential program for people with a dual diagnosis of serious mental illness and substance abuse, a supported housing program, an inpatient psychiatric hospital, and others. In many of these, I instituted or enhanced educational and support groups for families. Since 1980, I have also had a part-time private practice in Berkeley, California, where I have seen a variety of individual clients and families. In addition, I have provided training for families and for professionals in the United States and Canada.

Ways of thinking about and working with families who have a relative with mental illness have changed enormously since I began working in the field. Prior to the 1980s, families themselves were often assumed to be directly responsible for a relative's schizophrenia or affective disorder. There was a prevalent belief that faulty family interaction caused the illness and that therapy was therefore the most effective treatment.

Today, the predominant medical thinking holds that these illnesses have a significant physiological component. The chaos and disruption in the family result from the fact that a family member is disabled by an illness that the family cannot understand and that he or she has symptoms that are bizarre, confusing, unpredictable, and, at times, frightening.

A study in 1979 by Agnes Hatfield, a well-known educator and the mother of a son with a mental illness, concluded that what families actually want and need is very different from what mental-health professionals thought they wanted and needed. Families need education about the illnesses, specific suggestions for coping with their relative's behavior, and the support and empathy that comes from relating to other people facing similar experiences. In my work with hundreds of different families who have a relative with a mental illness, I have seen that when such families are offered these things, their lives are significantly improved and they are enormously grateful.

Over many years of teaching classes and leading educational support groups, I am consistently moved by the responses of families who report that what they learn has a significant impact on their lives and on those of other family members. Typical responses include such statements as: "Family education such as this should be required by law following diagnosis"; "The class was especially valuable in helping me be more detached, patient, understanding, and willing to still hang in there when I thought I couldn't anymore"; "I wish this had been available years ago."

Much of the material in this book I first developed for classes I taught in a variety of settings.

HOW TO USE THIS BOOK

The book as a whole serves as an introductory course on serious mental illnesses and how to deal with them. The first two chapters provide the basic background information necessary to understand schizophrenia and major affective disorders as well as the current forms of treatment. The rest of the book focuses on how to handle day-to-day interactions with people with a mental illness.

Chapter 3 provides an overview of general guidelines and basic skills necessary for successful interactions and communication with people who have a mental illness.

Chapter 4 explains how to handle psychotic symptoms (hallucinations, delusions, and disorganized speech). This is what families and friends most want to know. ("What do I say when I pick up the phone and the operator tells me there is a collect call from Jesus Christ? I know it's my son and I feel angry and embarrassed.") We also talk about handling ill persons' anger and how to help them manage stress and minimize relapses.

Chapter 5 focuses on dealing with even more severe and disconcerting symptoms: bizarre behavior, violence, substance abuse, and suicide.

In chapter 6 we turn our attention to helping families and friends deal with all the feelings they inevitably experience as a result of having a relative disabled by a mental illness. Whether you are a child embarrassed by your ill mother's behavior, a sibling angry at your family for focusing on your ill brother, or a parent guilt-ridden by your inability to ameliorate your child's pain, you will learn that you are not alone in how you feel. It is of prime importance that families and friends make the most of their own lives in spite of the special burdens they bear.

Chapter 7 explores the challenge of balancing the needs of the ill person with the needs of other family members. We present ways to make the time you spend with your ill relative as enjoyable as possible, as well as family problem-solving techniques. The painful and difficult question of whether the ill relative should live at home is also addressed.

Chapter 8 goes on to provide a brief overview of the mental-health system, describing the professionals and facilities that work with people with mental illness. We offer advice on how to best handle and work with professionals and facilities.

Chapter 9 focuses on handling external and practical matters such as what to say to friends or coworkers about your relative's illness. We discuss how to handle financial matters involving ill persons as well as how to help them find suitable housing and employment (if they are able to do so). Dealing with the ignorance, prejudice, and stigma you will encounter all along the way is discussed as well.

The Quick Reference Guides in this book can be used as instant reminders of how to deal with specific issues or situations when they arise. I encourage you to read through the book and then use the Quick Reference Guides to assist you in your day-to-day interactions with your loved one.

Added in the revised edition is important material about substance abuse, now an enormous problem for people with mental illness. In the concluding chapter there is also a discussion of recovery, both from mental illness and from addiction.

Introduction to the Revised Edition

Many things have changed in the past ten years, since writing the first edition of this book. Most notably on the bright side, the public has been gradually gaining greater understanding of mental illness. This was dramatically illustrated in 2002 when *A Beautiful Mind* won the Academy Award for Best Picture. For the first time there was a compassionate portrayal of a person with schizophrenia in a leading role. NAMI (formerly National Alliance for the Mentally Ill) has succeeded in getting some states to pass "parity" laws that require medical insurance coverage of mental illness to be equal to that of other illnesses. Many new medications are now available, assisting tens of thousands of people with serious mental illness to have a better quality of life.

The possibility of recovering from mental illness is one of the most exciting and positive concepts developed in the past ten years. It comes primarily from people who have learned to live productive lives despite major psychiatric disorders. Consumers of mental-health services have become more active and organized, and have done a great deal to empower themselves and to improve the mental-health service system. They have advocated a change in the language used to describe people who have serious mental illnesses. Many people prefer the term "consumer" for one who utilizes mental-health services. Others support the terms "ex-patient," "survivor," "client," or "individual." What must be avoided are terms that define a person by his or her illness, such as "a schizophrenic," "mental patient," or one of the "mentally ill." These tend to dehumanize people. It is crucial to view people first and foremost as human beings, who have strengths, goals, feelings, and skills, and who deserve—as everyone does—to be treated with respect and dignity.

On the other hand, statistics show an increase in the percentage of people with serious mental illnesses who also have severe problems with drugs and alcohol. Research shows that at least half to three quarters of people with a serious mental illness have co-occurring substance-abuse problems. It is extremely painful and complicated for family, friends, and caregivers to cope with such people. There is a glaring absence of material available to assist family and friends in dealing with people who have co-occurring substance-use and major psychiatric disorders.

Many people undergoing substance-abuse programs also have co-occurring mental illness or post-traumatic stress disorders that go untreated, thus making it extraordinarily difficult for such individuals to remain clean and sober after leaving programs. Unfortunately, the mental-health and substance-abuse service systems have not yet found their way to full integration. Consumers continue to ping-pong from one system to the other despite growing research indicating that treating both problems concurrently is most effective. While there are a few good dual diagnosis programs and services scattered around the United States, there exists only a small fraction of what is needed.

There is an enormous amount of information that family, friends, and caregivers need when someone they care about has what is now referred to as "co-occurring disorders," or a dual diagnosis of a major psychiatric disorder plus a substance-use disorder. Caregivers need to learn not only all about substance abuse but also about the complex interaction of substance use with symptoms of major psychiatric disorders and with psychiatric medications.

It is somewhat misleading to use one term to describe all people with both major psychiatric disorders and substance-use disorders. The fact is that there is a great deal of variation among people who struggle with both problems. Some researchers and providers divide those with co-occurring disorders into one of four groups: one group consists of people with severe symptoms of both disorders; another includes individuals with less severe disorders; and the other two groups are made up of those with one severe disorder and the other less so. People with "less severe" psychiatric disorders are those whose primary psychiatric diagnosis is a personality disorder, an anxiety disorder, or a condition other than the ones addressed in this book. Here we are speaking chiefly of people who have schizophrenia, bipolar disorder, schizoaffective disorder, or severe, medication-resistant major depression.

The treatment and family coping strategies most effective for people with "less severe" psychiatric disorders are somewhat different from those presented here. "Less severe" is in quotes to acknowledge that people with a primary diagnosis of a personality disorder or other psychiatric conditions also have many serious problems with which to contend. Their families and caregivers need education and support to learn how best to cope with the issues they face. Just as one program cannot successfully serve all people, neither can one book provide the advice needed for those in all four groups.

Whether someone has a more or less severe substance-use problem will guide the kinds of interventions used, either more geared to substance-use problems or toward psychiatric disorders. Substance-use disorders, like major psychiatric disorders, are not constant. Typically, there are periods where the substance use is more active and other times when psychiatric symptoms are more acute. Caregivers need to learn two sets of interventions and to determine which to use or to modify in particular instances. This is a very difficult assessment even for trained staff to make.

The World of Mental Illness

*I*N ORDER TO HAVE compassion for people with mental illness, we must understand that they are suffering from symptoms or experiences that are largely beyond their control. Their thoughts and feelings may bounce around within them in illogical and unpredictable ways. They are at least as terrified by these experiences as we may be by their actions.

The lives of people with mental illness are made much more difficult by the fact that most people do not understand them. Often they are feared, avoided, or mocked. The alienation, isolation, and depression they feel as a result of these attitudes become secondary symptoms of the illness and make their lives more painful.

SCHIZOPHRENIA

Schizophrenia is a thought disorder, meaning that its main symptoms have to do with disturbance in thinking. For a person with schizophrenia, when symptoms are present the ability to think (and therefore to talk) in a consistently clear, organized, logical, and realistic manner is seriously impaired.

The current medical understanding is that what we call schizophrenia is probably a group of disorders rather than a single specific one. Just as there are many different kinds of cancer, there appears to be a number of different kinds of schizophrenia. They have some common symptoms, respond similarly to certain treatments, and have somewhat predictable courses and outcomes, but there are still many differences.

Technically, to be diagnosed as having schizophrenia, people must meet three criteria: they must be psychotic for at least six months *and* exhibit a deteriorating level of functioning *and* have no other organic factor or substance use at cause to any large extent. A person who is having one of the internal experiences described below is considered to be psychotic. When a person's level of functioning deteriorates, it means that he or she is not able to maintain the level of work, social life, or self-care that he or she previously did. (Keep in mind that this is a matter of degree; the situation must become extreme to justify a diagnosis.)

Psychosis is often incorrectly thought to be the same as mental illness. However, psychosis is a primary symptom often exhibited by people with schizophrenia or major affective disorders. Other organic conditions—such as Alzheimer's disease, multiple sclerosis, senility, or advanced stages of alcoholism—can also produce psychosis. Anyone can experience a *substance-induced psychosis* by taking certain drugs, or a *brief reactive psychosis* by being traumatized by an extremely horrible situation or deprived of sleep for many days. Psychotic symptoms also will occur if certain parts of the brain are stimulated by electrodes.

A person who is psychotic experiences one or more of three basic symptoms: hallucinations, delusions, and disorganized speech. Since these symptoms may be a recurring part of the lives of most people with schizophrenia and severe affective disorders, it is important that they be well understood.

Hallucinations

A *hallucination* is any sensory experience that is not caused by an external reality. Any one of our five senses—sight, sound, smell, taste, and touch—can be the focus of a hallucination. A person can hear voices that do not exist; he or she can see things that are not there, smell things when no odor is present, or feel things, like bugs crawling up his or her arms, when nothing is touching him or her. What is most important to understand about hallucinations is that they feel as real to the person having them as the words on this page seem to you.

Hearing voices is the most common kind of hallucination experienced by people with schizophrenia. Over time the voices often become insulting and demeaning to the ill person. The voices may also tell the person to do things that are inappropriate or dangerous. Sometimes the voices are entertaining and cause the ill person to smile or burst out laughing at seemingly inappropriate times.

People who suffer from hallucinations are often very confused and frightened by them. Some people learn to recognize that these experiences are different from the reality that others share, that they are experiencing a symptom of their illness and must try to prevent it from influencing what they do. Others, unfortunately, are never able to come to such an understanding. They believe that what they hear or see is real and true. For these people, life becomes a great deal more difficult because they must find a way to integrate what their voices are telling them with other, often contradictory, experiences. For example, a voice may tell a son that his father tried to poison him. This information is difficult to reconcile with the loving interactions the son usually has with his father.

Delusions

A *delusion* is a false belief. Many people with schizophrenia believe that the people they see on television are talking directly to them. People who are delusional truly believe things that we know to be obviously untrue. People with paranoid schizophrenia typically believe that others are trying to harm them. Many others have delusions with religious themes. They may believe that they are Jesus Christ or that they must do certain, perhaps bizarre, things because God wants them to.

One of the most important things to know about people who are delusional is that they will not change their beliefs if you tell them they are delusional. This would be like a person telling you that you are not who you think you are but someone else entirely, and expecting you to believe it.

Disorganized Speech

Speech may be disorganized in a variety of ways. The person may "slip off track," jumping from one topic to another. Answers to questions may be only vaguely related, completely unrelated, or nearly incomprehensible. Disorganized speech is a reflection of extremely disturbed thinking and impairs the ability to communicate effectively. It is far more extreme than the way many of us become in the heat of an upsetting or stressful situation.

For example, a woman who is psychotic may try to explain to you that the way the Brooklyn Bridge is built is absolute proof that the Democrats ought to be in power. She may explain in great detail about how the bridge was constructed and about what Democrats believe in. She may go on to tell you how she is happy because she is sad and tired. While each sentence may be grammatically correct, the discussion as a whole makes no sense. This can be further confusing to families when, an hour later, the same woman does a good job of preparing lunch and has a coherent conversation about it.

Inappropriate Affect

One of the next most common symptoms of schizophrenia, *inappropriate affect,* becomes apparent when the feelings someone displays do not fit with the content of his or her speech. An example of this is the woman who laughs as she talks of the death of a loved one, or is disappointed when she hears about a victory for her favorite team. The feelings of people with inappropriate affect also often seem to change rapidly for no apparent reason. One moment they may be laughing and the next crying, with the listener unable to figure out what was so funny in the first place. Such a person is described as being *labile.*

One of the most disconcerting things about these symptoms is that they are not usually present all the time. They will typically come and go from hour to hour and day to day; sometimes they will be absent for weeks or even months in people with a serious mental illness.

MAJOR AFFECTIVE DISORDERS

In major affective disorders the main symptoms have to do with disturbances of *mood.* Moods are disturbed if they are too up (manic) or too down (depressed), or if they alternate between the two. The two most common major affective disorders are *bipolar disorder* (formerly called manic depression) and *major depressive disorder.* In bipolar disorder people at times experience episodes of feeling manic and at other times episodes of feeling depressed. In major depressive disorder people have periods of extreme depression only. In both bipolar and major depressive disorders people also experience periods when their moods are relatively normal. The patterns vary enormously from one person to another as far as how long the episodes last and how frequently they occur. Over time, however, regular patterns usually develop with each individual.

Many of us know people we consider moody. This, however, is very different from their having an affective disorder. To warrant a diagnosis of any of the serious affective disorders, the moods must be extreme. The depression must be so severe that a person's eating or sleeping patterns are seriously disturbed or the person is so lacking in energy or interest that he or she can barely do anything at all. Feelings of worthlessness, hopelessness, and helplessness abound. Severely depressed people may have great difficulty concentrating and making decisions. They may feel so bad that they think about suicide.

A depression can also reach a psychotic level when the feelings lead to delusional thinking (believing things that are not true). An example of this is the depressed woman who, thinking she is responsible for the last major earthquake, becomes convinced that she should be put to death.

People in a manic state have moods that are so elevated that they often do quite inappropriate things. They talk in a fast-paced, pressured manner, their thoughts racing from one idea to another. They tend to sleep little, and their eating patterns may change significantly. They often spend enormous amounts of money (which they may not have) or give away many of their possessions. They are easily distracted, and their thinking may for periods of time be as disturbed as that of a person with schizophrenia. They may have grandiose delusions, believing that they are superhuman or have supernatural powers, leading to their engaging in dangerous or pleasurable activities, such as going on shopping sprees or having sex, to such excess that the consequences to themselves or their relationships are often quite negative.

OTHER DIAGNOSES

The American Psychiatric Association's official manual of diagnoses and classifications is known as the *Diagnostic and Statistical Manual of Mental Disorders*. With each periodic revision the number in the title changes. The fourth revised edition is therefore called D.S.M. IV. It would lead us to believe that all people with a serious mental illness fall into a clearly defined category. Unfortunately, life is not quite so clear-cut. There are many people who have some symptoms of schizophrenia and/or some symptoms of a serious affective disorder, yet do not fully meet the criteria for either one. These people may qualify for a diagnosis of schizoaffective disorder, schizophreniform disorder, borderline personality disorder with psychotic features, or any of several other more general diagnoses.

Ultimately the most significant consideration is which treatment or medication ought to be tried first. This might be of even greater importance if the medications and treatments available were completely effective, but they are not. Suffice it to say that if your relative has received several different diagnoses, you ought not be surprised or alarmed because:

- The symptoms people exhibit and experience may change over time.

- A doctor who does not know a patient over a long period of time can base a diagnosis only on what he or she sees and whatever history may be available to him or her.

- Doctors are not perfectly consistent in the way they diagnose people, especially those patients who exhibit a variety of symptoms.

- Some doctors have preferences for a particular diagnosis. Some countries also tend to lean toward certain diagnoses. In England, for example, people are more often diagnosed as manic-depressive, while in the United States a diagnosis of schizophrenia is more common.

THE SUBJECTIVE EXPERIENCE
OF MENTAL ILLNESS

Thus far I have described the symptoms of the major mental illnesses—schizophrenia and major affective disorders—as they may appear to a doctor viewing them from the outside. We must also understand what the symptoms feel like to a person who is having these unusual and often terrifying experiences. Only by understanding what a person with a mental illness is going through can you learn how to relate to that person and how to make your interactions with him or her more satisfying.

Feelings of Fear and Confusion

Fear dominates the lives of most people with mental illness, who live in perpetual dread of the onset of their next episode. They are also terrified of many things that seem il-logical or irrational. Their fear makes a good deal of sense when we consider how irrational and unpredictable their internal worlds are. They suddenly hear bizarre voices telling them absurd things. They may feel happy one moment and be crying the next for reasons they cannot explain. Their thoughts often race and their feelings rapidly change in the most frightening and unusual ways. Imagine what you might feel if you were listening to a radio while having the television on, with a ten-piece band playing in the background. Or imagine experiencing waves of sadness about a loved one who has recently died and then immediately hearing someone you cannot see telling you the funniest joke you've heard in years.

People with active symptoms of schizophrenia, and people in a manic state, are fairly consistently overstimulated by their own internal chaos and confusion. Some people with schizophrenia react to these stimuli by withdrawing into their own quiet place. They feel even more confused and overwhelmed when they are around people, especially larger groups. Others with schizophrenia try to drown out the noise and commotion inside themselves by playing loud music or going to places full of people and energy.

People with active schizophrenia say that much of the time their lives feel like a dream—and they mean that literally. If we think of our own nighttime dreams, we may get a glimpse of what their world is like. There, things happen without the usual logical progression. In our dreams, we may be peacefully swimming in a lake when suddenly an elephant is chasing us down the street. Time, place, and even our own identity can change without notice.

This internal chaos makes it difficult for people with mental illness to pay attention to our requests and may cause them to be unable to answer even as seemingly simple a question as "How are you today?" Whether such experiences are occasional, as they are for some people with schizophrenia, or common, as they are for others, people with schizophrenia experience life differently from the rest of us. The world most of us inhabit is simple by comparison: no fairy queens or wildly unpredictable feelings, visions, or thoughts to contend with. Just day-to-day life: work, family, friends, good times and bad—all of it making some kind of basic sense. Many people with schizophrenia rarely have such experiences.

All of this fear and chaos contributes to the limited ability of people with mental illness to concentrate, to learn, to solve problems, and to remember things. It also contributes to their seeming preoccupation with things others don't understand or notice, their inability to behave in socially acceptable ways, and their poor judgment. It may also explain the tendency many people with a mental illness have to be extremely impulsive. While this most substantial list of problems would be more than enough for anyone, it is only the beginning for people with mental illness.

A Confused Sense of Self

Many people with a serious mental illness also experience a symptom that professionals call *poor ego boundaries*. This translates into a profound confusion about where they end and others begin. They are very unclear, often without knowing it, about who is thinking or feeling what. For example, if your son with schizophrenia is angry about what he has just heard on the radio and you walk into his room, it may seem to him that you are angry. If your daughter with schizophrenia feels bad about not being able to work, she may yell at you for accusing her of being incompetent. She may feel sad and ask you why you are sad. If you give voice to something she just thought, she may accuse you of stealing her thoughts.

Feelings of Being Out of Control

A related and very common delusion of people with schizophrenia is that their minds are being controlled by someone or something outside of them. This may be the television or radio, beings from outer space, the FBI, a former friend, a doctor, a medication, and so forth. Any of these may be experienced as putting thoughts in their minds (thought insertion), of taking their ideas away (thought withdrawal), or of radiating their thoughts (thought broadcasting).

This makes some sense if we consider how little control people with schizophrenia have over their thinking. Anyone whose thoughts were racing and changing at random, and who was unable to stop or even slow down the process, would likely feel that things were out of control and would begin to wonder who or what was creating such confusion.

A Tendency to Attribute Special Meaning to Events

People who have a mental illness can be so confused in their thinking that you can never predict how they will interpret things you say and do. Certain words or actions may have a special significance to them. Similarly, they may feel compelled to perform certain rituals in order to feel safe.

On the face of it these behaviors may seem bizarre and absurd. However, they do make some sense when you consider that humans need order and logic. Because there is little of either in the lives of people who are afflicted with a mental illness, they devise new and unusual ways to make sense of their constantly unpredictable experiences.

Ideas of Reference

People with a serious mental illness often experience a symptom called *ideas of reference*—feelings that much of what happens is, somehow, related to them. These people feel that many moves other people make, from scratching their heads to selling their houses, may be done because of something the ill person did or said. Or a gesture may be interpreted as a secret signal intended to control what the ill person will do or feel.

These experiences are often misinterpreted as self-centeredness or an inflated sense of self on the part of the ill person. Ideas of reference are not easily corrected or controlled by the ill person or anyone treating him or her, when medication is ineffective or not taken. Then the best that can be done is to help the person learn, over time, that such ideas are one of his or her symptoms, and do not always reflect the way things really are. Some people can never learn this.

Loose Associations

People with mental illness will often associate one idea or word with another that may have only a loose connection to the first. In clinical terms, they are making *loose associations*. For example, a young woman with schizophrenia may start out talking about what she *saw* in the paper, then switch to what kind of *saw* she used to cut wood, then move on to what she *would* like to have for dinner. It is difficult, and at times impossible, to follow the connections that people with mental illness are making when they talk, think, or write. This causes communication with them to be quite a challenge.

Hypersensitivity to Criticism

For reasons no one fully understands, people with a serious mental illness will often remember negative comments more easily than positive ones. This means that, for example, if you tell your son with a mental illness something he did well and something he did poorly when he cleaned his room yesterday, he will likely remember only what he did wrong. This has some important ramifications in terms of how to effectively give praise and criticism to people with a mental illness (see chapter 3).

Despair and Loss of Energy

People who have severe depressions feel miserable. They have no energy. They have no interest in doing anything. They feel immobilized. They often feel unable to get out of bed or to feed or dress themselves. Paying a bill seems an overwhelming task. They often cannot remember ever feeling any better and have no hope that they will feel better in the future. Life seems meaningless. They feel completely unable to do anything to make themselves feel better. In addition, many believe that there is some reason they are feeling so bad—that they must have done something to deserve such punishment.

Capacity for Insight

There is a great deal of variation in the symptoms and personal characteristics that people with mental illness exhibit. This also applies to the ability of such people to have insight into their illness and behavior. Some people can be taught that they are ill and that they need to take medication and participate in treatment; they can learn how to recognize their symptoms and how to tell when their symptoms are getting better or worse.

Others never seem able to learn any of this; life becomes much more difficult for them. They are unable to benefit from their own experiences, no matter how painful these may be. For example, the fact that your mother twice ended up in jail or a hospital after running down the street naked for some delusional reason (perhaps believing that God wanted her to do so) may not stop her from doing this a third time and even a fourth. How to interact most effectively with people who lack insight into their illness is discussed further in chapter ten.

It is important to understand and recognize all the symptoms described above because they are so easily misinterpreted as manipulation or uncooperativeness. What makes mental illnesses so difficult to live with is the fact that symptoms can come and go with no apparent reason. These illnesses are cyclical in nature, and the cycles may be longer and more severe for some people than for others. Someone may seem to be doing better for a period of time (and relatives may get their hopes up), and then the symptoms return (causing everyone to be devastated or infuriated).

We must learn to enjoy the good times, and to get through the bad times as best we can. It does no one any good to get angry or disappointed with the ill person for not being able to prevent a relapse when we, with all our medical knowledge, are unable to do so. Rather, we must direct our anger and frustration at the illness. This takes time, education, and experience.

SECONDARY SYMPTOMS OF MENTAL ILLNESS

Our discussion thus far has focused on the primary symptoms of schizophrenia and major affective disorders—that is, those symptoms that occur as a direct result of having the illnesses. There are also secondary symptoms. To make an analogy, the primary symptom of having a broken arm is that you cannot move your arm. Secondary symptoms may be that you cannot go to work and you feel angry and depressed that your life is less productive and less exciting while your arm is healing.

The secondary symptoms of having a serious mental illness in this country are profound. While there have long been campaigns to educate people about cancer, AIDS, and drug and alcohol abuse, these have only recently taken place for schizophrenia and affective disorders. In fact, most people still do not understand mental illnesses. As a result, many are afraid of those with a mental illness or think such people are weird; in either case, they want nothing to do with them. This leaves people with a mental illness not only disabled by their symptoms, but isolated and rejected by others. They may therefore feel alienated, empty, lonely, rejected, and depressed. As a result of this, they often withdraw from people and activities, lose interest in the world, and become mistrustful. They may feel increasingly angry or bitter—and they have good reason to be: life is more limited and difficult for them. Many of their childhood dreams and hopes may never be realized.

The fact that many people with mental illness wind up feeling hopeless, betrayed, or cheated is not difficult to understand. One unfortunate consequence of these feelings is that many of these people ultimately wind up killing themselves. While people with a mental illness are no more violent than anyone else, they are more likely to commit suicide.

About 10 percent of those with schizophrenia and severe bipolar disorder ultimately end their own lives. Some do so in the middle of a psychotic episode, perhaps not believing they will really die. Many do so out of the pain of living a life that feels so empty, isolated, and limited that it seems no longer worth continuing.

CAUSES OF MENTAL ILLNESS

Once you have some understanding of what the major mental illnesses are, the next questions you are likely to ask are "What causes them?" and "Who is likely to get them?" Unfortunately, the answers to these crucial questions are still surrounded by many myths and misunderstandings.

Until relatively recently, the methods available for studying the brain were fairly limited, consisting primarily of performing autopsies on the brains of people who donated their bodies for research. This technique has obvious limitations: it is difficult to study how the brain works when it is dead.

The sophisticated devices that have recently become available have geometrically increased our understanding of the brain. Magnetic resonance imaging (MRI) scans give amazingly detailed information about the structure of the brain. They show physical abnormalities within the brain and indicate the presence of tumors. Improvements in computer and radiation technology have made MRI pictures far more informative than their ancestors—X rays and CT (computed tomography) scans.

Ways of studying the functioning of the brain have been similarly revolutionized by the development of techniques that measure the metabolism of glucose and oxygen in the brain. When this information is combined with a positron emission tomography (PET) scan, it is possible to generate

three-dimensional pictures of the brain while it is involved
in various activities. Clear differences in the functioning of
the brains of so-called normal people as compared with the
functioning of the brains of those with schizophrenia or
Alzheimer's can be seen. Although this is all exciting and interesting, it leaves unanswered many questions about what
causes mental illnesses and how to prevent or cure them.

Geneticists have also made enormous contributions to
our pool of knowledge about mental illnesses. They have located key chromosomes and genetic markers in people who
have bipolar disorders; they can trace these on family trees.
Yet all this information can provide neither a way to determine whether a person has an illness before symptoms develop nor a way to prevent or cure the illnesses.

Ultimately, even considering these vastly improved techniques and our relative wealth of knowledge, what we do not
know about mental illness far outweighs what we do know.
While the technology developed in recent decades has made
remarkable breakthroughs possible, we still have a long way
to go: no one yet knows exactly what causes mental illnesses,
how to cure them, or how to predict in whom they will develop. We are therefore left to make certain deductions about
causes, treatment, and course of the illnesses based primarily
on observation of people who are ill, and on their family histories.

While some professionals still disagree, most now believe
that heredity is the most important factor in determining who
is likely to develop schizophrenia or major affective disorders. The evidence for the role of heredity is quite substantial:
Dr. E. Fuller Torrey, in his book *Surviving Schizophrenia,* presents convincing statistics, as do most other basic books about
schizophrenia. The chance of your getting schizophrenia depends upon how many, and which, of your relatives have it or
have had it.

- If no one in your family has ever had schizophrenia, you have a 1 percent chance of getting it. (This appears to be the occurrence of the illness in the general population.)
- If one second-degree relative (cousin, grandparent, and so forth) has it, you have about a 2 percent chance of getting it.
- If a first-degree relative (parent, brother, or sister) has it, your chances jump to about 10 percent.
- If both of your parents have it, the chances go up to about 40 percent.
- If you have an identical twin with it, you then have a 50 percent chance of becoming ill.
- If several relatives have it, add up the percentages that go with each relative to get a rough estimate. For example, if your father (10 percent) and a cousin (2 percent) are ill, you have about a 12 percent chance of getting schizophrenia.

Environment and child-rearing practices have often been thought to cause mental illness. The above statistics could also be interpreted as evidence for this connection, but additional data from other studies have shown heredity to be the major factor. These studies involved following the histories of children whose biological parents had schizophrenia and who were adopted by people who did not have schizophrenia. The number of these children who went on to develop schizophrenia was compared with the corresponding number in another group of adopted children, who were born to non-schizophrenic parents but were adopted by persons who had schizophrenia. The outcome statistics favor biology, not the environment: 10 percent of those born to a parent with schizophrenia developed the illness themselves even though they were raised by normal parents; 1 percent of those born to normal parents and raised by parents with schizophrenia developed the illness.

Studies of identical twins provide further evidence that biological factors rather than environmental ones determine the likelihood of a person's developing a serious mental illness. Identical twins who were adopted and raised separately were studied. Still about 50 percent of those whose twins developed schizophrenia developed the illness themselves.

There has been far less debate about the cause of major affective disorders. For decades mental-health professionals have agreed that the primary cause of affective disorders is physiological. This unanimity has provided some comfort to the families of people with affective disorders.

Families of people with schizophrenia, however, have been done an enormous disservice by, and have suffered much abuse from, professionals who believe that the behavior of the families, rather than a physiological factor, causes the illness. It is quite common to hear stories of families going to psychiatrists in hope of finding answers, understanding, and relief from the pain and suffering they and their ill relative are experiencing. Instead, they encounter doctors who either harshly tell them that they are to blame for their relative's condition, or refuse to talk to them at all. Families come away from these encounters more devastated, confused, and guilt-ridden than before.

Extensive research continues to be done. Scientists are exploring chemical imbalances in the brain, the functioning of neurotransmitters, the effects of viral infections (particularly during the second trimester of pregnancy), the blood flow to the brain and the enlargement of certain ventricles, and the atrophy of parts of the brain in people with schizophrenia.

There is, additionally, a good deal of evidence about what *does not* cause mental illness. Many families think that drugs and alcohol caused their relative to become ill. While the abuse of these substances is not helpful to people with a mental illness, there is no indication that they can cause the illnesses. There are millions of people who abuse drugs and alcohol and yet never develop any signs of schizophrenia or major affective disorder. It seems likely that people who are beginning to experience symptoms of mental illness turn to illegal drugs or alcohol to escape their discomfort and fear. This can further confuse and complicate the picture, because some drugs, such as PCP, can cause brain damage and symptoms similar to those of schizophrenia and bipolar disorder.

Similarly, no substantial evidence exists indicating that bad parenting, poor diet, lack of exercise, or vitamin deficiencies cause mental illnesses. While it is preferable for everyone to live a healthy life, abstain from drug abuse, eat well, and get enough sleep and exercise, many people who do only some or none of these never develop a mental illness. Conversely, when people are suffering from the symptoms of serious mental illness, exercising, taking care of personal hygiene, and eating well can seem like major accomplishments; performing any part of any of these tasks may be more than they can handle. Delusions or hallucinations can also affect what the person will do or eat.

STRESS

There is one external factor that is important to consider when discussing the causes of mental illnesses: *stress*. Stress does not cause these illnesses. However, it appears to increase the seriousness of the symptoms in people who are prone to the disorders. Many people can be subjected to extraordinary stress and never develop a mental illness. If, however, you are prone to the disorders, you are likely to be more sensitive to stress. Stress may be one factor in determining when the symptoms get better or worse.

Thus it is important for families and friends of people with a mental illness to become educated both about the illnesses and the effects of stress on the symptoms. While families do not cause and cannot cure the illnesses, they *can* significantly alter the level of stress in their relative's life. In this way, families and friends can play an important role in decreasing the severity of the symptoms and in minimizing the times when their ill relatives become so sick that they require hospitalization.

Note that stress can be anything that makes a person feel anxious or upset. An event that most of us would experience as completely insignificant, like answering the telephone or going to a restaurant, can be stressful for someone with a mental illness. We must learn what a particular person with a mental illness experiences as stressful and help find ways to reduce the stress. However, this does not mean that by doing so we can eliminate all symptoms or relapses, any more than by getting a sick person to drink fluids and rest we can cure the flu, although we may help minimize the severity.

MYTHS ABOUT MENTAL ILLNESS

Before moving on to the next chapter, which examines treatments for mental illness, I want to clearly present the truth behind eight common myths about mental illness.

MYTH: *Mental illness is very rare and unusual.*
FACT: Neither schizophrenia nor affective disorders are new or uncommon. Schizophrenia occurs in about 1 percent of the world's population, regardless of child-rearing practices, religion, socioeconomic status, race, political system, or any other variable. Some countries have a slightly higher incidence (for example, the Scandinavian countries and western

Ireland), while others have a slightly lower rate (for example, tropical Africa), for reasons that no one entirely understands. In the United States about 2.5 million people suffer from schizophrenia, and many more than that suffer from major affective disorders.

MYTH: *Some therapies can cure major mental illness.*
FACT: There is currently no known cure for schizophrenia or for major affective disorders. Some people claim to be able to cure select groups of people with mental illness. Their techniques, however, cannot be duplicated by others with a random group of people with mental illness. What we can do is reduce the severity of the symptoms in many people, and improve the quality of life for both those afflicted and their loved ones.

MYTH: *Having schizophrenia means having a split personality.*
FACT: Having schizophrenia does not mean having a split personality. The latter is a separate and very different psychiatric condition, technically called *dissociative identity disorder*. It is caused by repeated childhood traumas. People with this disorder (formerly called multiple personality disorder) go from one personality state to a dramatically different one. For example, a shy, socially awkward typist will periodically become an outgoing, seductive party hopper. He or she may have different names when in each different personality. The films *The Three Faces of Eve* and *Sybil* portray this disorder.

MYTH: *The mentally ill are violent.*
FACT: People with a mental illness are generally not violent—nor are they psychotic killers, as the media frequently portrays them. There is no higher incidence of violence among people with mental illness than among the population in general. This common myth has done a great disservice to people suffering from schizophrenia, most of whom are very withdrawn and quiet.

MYTH: *Mental illness is contagious.*
FACT: Mental illness is not contagious. You cannot catch it by spending time with, or drinking from the same glass as, someone who has it. You may briefly feel confused after spending time with someone who cannot think or talk clearly. However, after leaving that person and spending time with a clear-thinking adult, your confusion will disappear. It is like spending time with a child: although you begin to see and experience the world through the child's eyes, you are no closer to being a child afterward.

MYTH: *The mentally ill are bad or evil.*
FACT: People who have a mental illness are not evil. The fact that individuals are afflicted with these disorders does not mean they or their families did something wrong or are bad people. Having such an illness is mainly a matter of bad luck, as is being born with diabetes, a propensity toward heart disease, or cancer. There is no reason to feel ashamed of the fact that any of these illnesses may run in your family. Yet many families with a relative who has a mental illness do feel a great deal of shame.

MYTH: *The mentally ill are morally weak.*
FACT: Having a mental illness is not a sign of weakness. People with a mental illness cannot stop their symptoms by trying harder any more than someone who has impaired hearing can hear better by trying harder to listen.

MYTH: *People with mental illness are creative geniuses.*
FACT: There is the same percentage of people with above-average intelligence among people who have a mental illness as among those who do not have a mental illness. The same holds for artistic, creative, and mechanical abilities and all other skills and talents.

2

Understanding Treatments and the Course of Mental Illness

WHILE THERE IS NO known cure for serious mental illnesses, various forms of treatment are available and can offer significant relief. For some fortunate people, these treatments can alleviate many or all symptoms and enable them to live relatively normal lives. For others less fortunate, the treatments offer little or no relief. The only way to determine whether a treatment will help your relative is to go through the often long and painful process of trial and error. Why some people are helped by the treatments and others are not is an unknown. No one can predict who will or will not be helped. Success is probably related to individual physiological differences and to which type of illness a person has.

THE PRIMARY TREATMENT: MEDICATION

The single most effective form of treatment for most people with a major mental illness is medication. (I emphasize *single* here because the most effective overall treatment is a combination of medication and some type of social rehabilitation program or family living situation in which family members are educated and know how to use specific skills in dealing with the person with a mental illness.) There are, however, many disadvantages to medication, and many people have strongly negative feelings about it. While their resistance is understandable in some cases, medication is still the best single form of treatment currently available.

How effective medication is likely to be depends in part on what type of illness a person has and the severity of the symptoms. For some people the illness is so severe that they are completely disabled by the symptoms.

Affective disorders tend to respond to medication better than schizophrenia does, partly because they come in milder forms. Therefore, if your relative has a major depression or bipolar disorder, he or she has a better chance of being helped significantly by medication.

Many people with affective disorders live very full lives. They can work, have families and friends, and enjoy leisure activities. Many people with whom they have contact never know that they are taking medication or even that they suffer from a serious mental illness. In fact, there are many famous athletes, actors, and even some courageous politicians who have admitted to struggling with affective disorders. It is thought that Abraham Lincoln and Vincent Van Gogh suffered from manic depression. Those who have been open about their illness, such as Patti Duke and Lionel Aldridge (a former Green Bay Packer and star of the 1968 Super Bowl), have done a great deal to make this illness somewhat more respectable and acceptable to the world.

This has less often been the case for people with schizophrenia. Because they are often more seriously disabled by their illness, they have more difficulty representing themselves and reversing the attitudes of the public.

There are now several medications available for the treatment of bipolar disorder which are extremely effective in controlling symptoms. These are lithium and several antiseizure medications, such as those with the brand names of Depakote, Neurontin, and Tegretol. For approximately 80 percent of people with bipolar disorder these medications eliminate or minimize the mood swings—the ups or downs—that people with the disorder are prone to. About 20 percent of people with this illness, however, have very severe cases and are not helped much or at all by medication. Their lives are as difficult as are the lives of most people with schizophrenia. This is the group we refer to as people with severe manic-depression or severe bipolar disorder.

The other type of medication often given to people with affective disorders is antidepressants. As their name suggests, these help to improve depressed moods. When they work, which is to say when people are lucky enough that their bodies respond to them in the best possible way, the people taking them feel less depressed. Sometimes they feel they are back to normal.

There are many different kinds of antidepressants, manufactured by many different companies, and the same medication may have one or two different trade names. This is confusing to many people with a mental illness and to their families. In the Appendix I seek to clarify some of this information.

The news is not quite so good for people with schizophrenia. While about 80 percent do respond to the medications available for this illness, the response is often not as good. That is, the antipsychotic medications are not able to help these people as much as mood stabilizers help most people with bipolar disorder.

Medications may reduce psychotic symptoms somewhat or, occasionally, entirely. For example, someone who is plagued by voices may hear them more faintly, less often, or not at

all. A man with delusions may no longer believe that someone is trying to control his mind or that he is Peter Rabbit.
Some of the medications also have a sedative effect, helping
to calm the agitation people with schizophrenia often feel.
Some of the irrational and very changeable feelings described
in chapter 1 may also be reduced with such medications. Other
symptoms of schizophrenia, called the *negative symptoms,*
including lack of emotional or verbal responsiveness, poor
self-care and lack of motivation, were not helped by traditional antipsychotics, such as Thorazine and Haldol. They
are helped by newer medications, such as Risperdal, Zyprexa,
and Geodon.

There are many kinds of antipsychotic medications for
people who exhibit such symptoms as hallucinations, delusions, and confused thinking. Antipsychotic medications may
also be called major tranquilizers, neuroleptics, or phenothi-
azines. The list in the Appendix covers the antipsychotic drugs
commonly used. The older medications are called typical or
traditional antipsychotics and the newer ones "atypical."

Because medication reduces some of the primary symptoms, the secondary ones may also be reduced. People may be
able to concentrate better. They may feel more willing and
able to interact with others and to participate in low-stress
activities, to go to work, or to attend school. They also may
feel more comfortable engaging in other forms of treatment,
like social rehabilitation programs or psychotherapy.

Mood stabilizers, antidepressants, and antipsychotics often have undesirable effects, usually referred to as side effects.
These range from such mild effects as increased sensitivity to
the sun to such serious unpleasant effects as severe muscle
stiffness, extreme restlessness, blurred vision, and the involuntary movement of certain muscles.

In deciding whether to use a medication, positive effects

need to be weighed against the negative ones. This can be a difficult decision for even the most clear-thinking person. It is often an impossible one for someone with schizophrenia to make without the assistance of professionals and friends or family.

Fortunately, there are also medications to help reduce some of the unpleasant side effects. While these don't work all the time and even have some unpleasant side effects of their own, they can often help. Again, ill people and their families are faced with very complicated decisions and need to weigh the improvements that medications can bring against the complications involved in taking several medications.

Decisions about medications are particularly difficult because the therapeutic effects of medication sometimes take longer to be felt than do the side effects. For example, consider Tom, a young man with schizophrenia who believes that rays from the television are controlling him. His doctor and family want Tom to take medication. Getting a person like Tom to try medication in the first place is a major accomplishment. It will be even more difficult to persuade Tom that if he endures a few weeks of dry mouth and stiff muscles, he will begin thinking more clearly. (Keep in mind that such a person may not believe there is anything wrong with his or her thinking.) Now imagine the problems that can occur if that medication does not work well and it is recommended that Tom try another. This means asking him to tolerate other unpleasant side effects for at least a few days so that he may experience some therapeutic effect.

Prescribing medication for people with mental illness is far from the exact science many psychiatrists would have us believe it is. It is often a hit-or-miss process; Depakote is tried first for bipolar disorder, and atypical antipsychotics for schizophrenia. If those do not work, lithium or traditional antipsychotics may be tried, or an antidepressant when there are signs of depression. If none of these medications work, there are others, such as Tegretol, that may offer some relief.

Getting People to Take Medication and Go to Treatment

Families and friends must often deal with their relative's refusal to take medication or to participate in any or all forms of treatment. To see someone you love refuse the help that you know will decrease his or her suffering can be as infuri-

---

WHY PEOPLE RESIST ACCEPTING THAT THEY ARE ILL AND RESIST TAKING MEDICATION

People resist accepting that they are ill because:

1. They are experiencing denial—a common first reaction to shocking or bad news such as a death or the diagnosis of a seriously disabling illness.

2. They are in pain due to the social stigma associated with mental illness. The implications for the future are also painful and involve:

   - grieving the loss of some of their dreams and the ability to have normal lives
   - lowering their expectations for what they will have in their lives
   - accepting the need for long-term treatment

3. They are experiencing a symptom of the illness, in one of several ways:

ating as it is heartbreaking. The first step in dealing with this situation is to step back and think about why the person is making such an irrational and seemingly self-defeating choice.

I have summarized several possible reasons in the Quick Reference Guide entitled Why People Resist Accepting That They Are Ill and Resist Taking Medication.

Note that I especially focus on two issues—one related to our social environment, the other to the illness itself. It is extremely difficult for many people to accept that they have a mental illness in our unsympathetic culture. They may expe-

---

- continued, massive denial of problems—a primitive defense mechanism to preserve the fragile sense of self-esteem that some ill people have
- delusional thinking, poor judgment, or poor reality testing

People resist taking medication because:

1. The side effects can be upsetting and unpleasant.
2. It may mean admitting that they have a mental illness.
3. It may feel like they are being controlled by an outside force. It can trigger issues people have about loss of power and control in their lives.
4. Reducing symptoms, and thus seeing the limitation of their lives, can be more painful than being lost in psychosis. Many people in manic episodes prefer that high-energy state to the lower-energy one they feel on medication.

rience shame, pain, and even greater depression. Accepting that you have a mental illness is no easy pill to swallow. It often means acknowledging that your life will be different than you had hoped. Some people believe that if they can survive without any type of treatment, it proves that they are not a *mental case.*

Other reasons are more directly related to symptoms of

GETTING THE ILL PERSON TO GO TO TREATMENT AND TAKE MEDICATION

Break large goals down into small steps and set up a realistic timetable. The pace will usually be much slower than you would prefer. Each individual goal can take months to reach. For example, in order to attend a day program one must be able to:

1. wake up on time
2. organize and prepare to leave home
3. use transportation
4. tolerate group interaction and social contact

Let your ill relative know that you have clear expectations that he or she will progress. Develop a system of rewards for each small step taken. Offer things such as acknowledgment and encouragement, special treats or privileges, and additional financial support. This creates an environment in which the person feels safe in trying new things. Do not dwell on failures or mistakes.

Refer to past experiences that may remind your

the illnesses. Remember, many of the symptoms interfere with the ability to think clearly and logically. People who have a serious mental illness may have all sorts of delusional reasons for not wanting to have anything to do with doctors, hospitals, programs, or medications. Some of these may contain a kernel of truth based on bad experiences they have had in treatment facilities.

relative of how much better his or her life was when he or she was taking medication or in treatment. Connect specific problems or negative consequences such as winding up in jail or the hospital to previous unsuccessful attempts to stop medication or treatment prematurely.

Familiarize yourself with the mental-health system as well as with programs and medication for people with mental illness. This allows you to be far more reassuring and realistic when your relative is ready to participate in a treatment program or take medication.

Deal with any ambivalence, doubts, sense of defeat, and so forth that you may have about treatments or medication. The chances are extremely high that these are somehow being conveyed to your relative and are having a negative impact on him or her.

Remember that the road to success is always a long and winding one, with many ups and downs. Expect a step or two backward to be interspersed with the forward ones.

Keep in mind that the benefits of the medication or treatment may eventually provide enough reward that your relative is willing to continue.

In chapter ten, there is further discussion of how to help people who lack insight into their illness. Those who are dead set against medications or treatment are unlikely to be persuaded by friends or family. In most parts of this country, it is now illegal to force adults to accept medication or treatment against their will, unless they are assessed as posing an imminent danger to themselves or others. The Quick Reference Guide entitled Getting the Ill Person to Go to Treatment and Take Medication outlines ways to help your relative achieve these goals.

One thing to remember while attempting to get someone to take medication or go to treatment is that the outcome is more important than the reasoning behind it. Some people will accept medication or treatment for as irrational a reason as others will refuse it. It is best not to argue with them. If they think the medication will help them become a world-class athlete, or that it is just sleeping pills, you would be wise not to discuss the matter further. Be grateful that they are willing to take the medication. Similarly, some people will see a psychiatrist or go to a program in order to help some other unfortunate souls or because they believe they are studying the profession. It is more important to praise them for going, to wish them well, and to hope they benefit from it than it is to argue the logic of their reasoning.

Accepting help may seem to you like a simple, obvious step for an ill person to take; in most cases this is not so. Usually you must help the person break the process down into small steps and devise a realistic timetable. Remember that before a person can take medication he or she must first be willing to talk to a doctor (who is the only one who can prescribe it). This in itself can take months, or even years.

Improving Medication Compliance

Some families have to deal with a slightly different problem: their relatives may be willing to take medication, but not consistently. Following are several suggestions that can help increase a person's willingness to take medication more regularly:

- *Listen carefully.* It is important that families, and doctors who prescribe medication, listen carefully and respond to the ill person's concerns, fears, or discomfort with the medication. The ill person needs to know that people are taking his or her concerns seriously. It is important, for instance, to acknowledge and confirm that the side effects may be uncomfortable.

- *Do not trivialize the discomfort.* Instead, remind the person that the benefits outweigh the discomfort, and that there are things that can be done to reduce the discomfort. For example, the person could drink more water for dry mouth, or use sunblock for increased sensitivity to the sun.

- *Provide education.* Help your relative learn as much as he or she can comfortably absorb about the medication. It is usually useful for people with a mental illness to know the positive effects of medication, as well as what happens when they do not take medication at all or when they take it inconsistently. They should also be made aware of all the possible side effects and how to deal with them.

- *Use the medication of choice.* If, for some rational or irrational reason, your relative prefers one equally effective medication over another, encourage that person to tell this to his or her doctor, who ideally will respect this preference.

- *Create a simple system.* Help your relative find a simple way to remember to take his or her medication. Sometimes people are so confused or distracted that they forget. Do not nag; just help the person remember. Be creative. Work with your relative to set up a chart, a daily pill box, a routine of taking medication before meals—whatever he or she prefers. Whatever works best is fine as long as there is a way for the person to know, each day, when to take the medication and whether he or she has indeed taken it.

- *Consider using injections.* Some medications come in long-acting injectable form. People need to get a shot only once or twice a month and don't have to think about medication the rest of the time. This procedure can make the medication process easier for some people. Others are afraid of needles and will avoid them like the plague.

- *Be supportive yet firm.* Give lots of praise when the responsibility is handled well. Taking medication can make such a difference in some people's lives that it may be worth your taking a strong stand. If other methods of improving compliance have not worked and your relative does significantly better when taking medication, you might follow the lead of some families and make it a condition for living at home or spending time with you.

One challenge families and friends repeatedly face is lowering their expectations and learning how to be patient. You and your relative will do much better when you shift your focus to the little steps that are taken from week to week. It is best for everyone involved not to dwell on long-term goals or possibilities. Let your goal be to help your relative live the best life he or she can *today and tomorrow.*

We all hope that someday treatments will offer new possibilities for people with mental illness. Until then, focusing on the present is the best approach. If your ill relative questions you about whether you think he or she will be able to do more next year or in five years, the best response is the most honest one. You have no way of knowing what the future will bring. Regardless of what history seems to suggest is most likely, scientists make new discoveries each year. You do not want to foster unrealistic hopes, yet you also do not want to feed despair about the future. Simply saying that you do not know what will happen, that you do not know whether he or she will ever be able to have a family, a job, or a car, is the best response. Then help the person refocus on the small steps to take today to work toward whatever long-term goals he or she has. You can assure such people that by taking small steps toward their goals, they can have more in their lives, and feel better about themselves, than they do today.

REHABILITATION PROGRAMS

The next most important kind of treatment for most people with schizophrenia or severe affective disorders is that offered by rehabilitation programs. Unfortunately, such programs are becoming increasingly scarce as federal and state funding for them is being slashed mercilessly. This is probably the second most tragic phenomenon that people suffering with a mental illness and their families have to deal with: the illnesses themselves bring more pain and heartache than any family deserves; to live in a country that has learned how to provide a wide range of useful services for people with mental illness and then to see that country choose to close those services is as infuriating as it is devastating.

Nonetheless, being familiar with the kinds of programs that do help can assist you in working toward their continued existence. Such services include social, vocational, and day programs; residential programs and inpatient hospitals; outpatient programs; and partial hospital programs. They may be called psychosocial rehabilitation, day treatment, socialization, case management, supported housing, or vocational training. We will discuss them further in chapter 8.

Whatever their form, there are several crucial functions that these programs serve:

- They may provide a structured, productive way for people to spend their time.

- They can educate people about their illness, symptoms, and medication and foster gradual acceptance of the illness and the limitations it imposes on them. Clients can learn techniques for managing and reducing disturbing symptoms. Different techniques (for example, ignoring the voices, telling the voices to leave, or going to a quiet place) are effective for different people.

- They provide a safe and supportive environment in which people with mental illness can talk about sensitive issues and try out different ways of dealing with their problems.

- They offer practice in basic social and living skills, such as shopping, cooking, using public transportation, and keeping a checking account. These tasks require initial training or review for those who knew the skills prior to becoming ill. Such programs go a long way toward combating the social isolation that plagues many people with mental illness. Clients in such programs can also learn how to better manage stress.

- They help people with mental illness develop realistic goals. Everyone needs to have goals in life. It is difficult for people with mental illness to figure out what they may realistically expect of themselves in the future.

In the best of all worlds, and with adequate funding, programs of various kinds would be available to all people with a serious mental illness. Support and education would be available to their families as well. However, since very few programs are currently in existence, families have increasingly become the primary caretakers and treaters. This is an enormous task, and families usually need special training and support.

OTHER TREATMENTS

There are three other kinds of treatments useful for people with a mental illness.

Talk Therapy

The most helpful type of talk therapy focuses on solving practical, day-to-day life problems: how to make friends, how to get along with family, how to deal with symptoms, and how to accept the illness and the limitations it brings. This kind of therapy, at its best, can help people put together the most satisfying life possible. The long-term, consistent relationship established with the therapist is often a rare and most valuable commodity in the lives of people with a serious mental illness. Remember that while talk therapy can help

people accept that they are ill and need medication and rehabilitation programs, it is not likely to reduce the symptoms
themselves.

Traditional Freudian psychoanalysis tends to raise people's anxiety and is not very useful for people with a serious
mental illness. It can even make some people so anxious that
they become more symptomatic.

Self-Help Groups

There are an increasing number of groups run and organized by clients and former patients. These self-help programs
range from centers offering many social and recreational activities to support groups that meet monthly or weekly, such
as Recovery Inc. Spending time with people who have similar
experiences and difficulties can provide comfort and connections that are to be found nowhere else. People who have a
mental illness are often able to learn and accept things from
their peers that professionals and families have been trying, in
vain, to tell them for years.

Electroconvulsive Therapy

More commonly referred to as shock treatment, electro-
convulsive therapy (ECT) has gotten a poor reputation over
the years. It is not an effective form of treatment for schizophrenia and has been misused as such in the past. It is, however, an effective form of treatment for people who have severe
depressions. In situations where antidepressant medication
has not worked, it is definitely worth considering. ECT has
been extremely valuable to many people who have been immobilized by depression. Modern techniques for administer-
ing ECT have made it a painless procedure.

MEASURING THE EFFECTIVENESS
OF TREATMENTS

Measuring the effectiveness of various kinds of treatments is a very difficult task when any long-term, serious, cyclical illness is involved. One of the simplest measurements is the relapse rate: how frequently people get so sick that they need to return to the hospital within a one-year period. While studies differ somewhat, they tend to suggest that the relapse rate for people with schizophrenia is likely to be about 70 percent with no treatment at all. This means about seven out of ten people with schizophrenia will need to return to the hospital within a year if they do not seek treatment. Taking antipsychotic medication and participating in no other form of treatment can bring the relapse rate down to about 30 percent. Any other form of treatment by itself does not significantly affect the relapse rate. When we combine medication with the specific kind of talk therapy described above, the relapse rate goes down to about 20 percent.

The best results are achieved, however, when we combine medication with participation in a social rehabilitation program. Then the relapse rate drops down to about 10 percent. The same is true when we combine medication with life in a family that has received training in how to deal with a relative who has a mental illness.

It seems fair to assume that as the relapse rate goes down, the quality of a person's life increases (though this is difficult to measure): he or she can spend time in more productive ways, get along better with other people, experience some happy times, and be tormented less by the symptoms of the illness.

SOME INEFFECTIVE TREATMENTS

There are numerous other forms of treatment that some people think are effective in treating serious mental illnesses, such as the use of high doses of vitamins (also called megavitamin therapy or orthomolecular psychiatry), changes in diet, the use of Dilantin, and psychoanalysis. However, most professionals who work with people with schizophrenia or major affective disorders believe that these approaches are not effective. Although some studies have suggested that these approaches work, when others try to duplicate the results they are unable to do so.

Another approach to psychosis encourages people to go into their delusions and fully experience their madness. This method may hold some value for healthier people who are experiencing some kind of life or identity crisis, but it tends to make people with a serious mental illness worse.

SELECTING A DOCTOR, THERAPIST, OR REHABILITATION PROGRAM

If you have a relative who is willing to see a doctor or therapist or to participate in a rehabilitation program, you are in a better starting position than many families. However, choosing people to work with your relative can be a confusing and complicated process.

Following are several guidelines to use when searching for a therapist for a relative or friend who has a mental illness.

- Get the name of a good therapist or doctor by word of mouth. Begin by asking people who might know of an appropriate person, such as a friend or relative of any-one who has been treated for a similar condition.

- Check with your local chapter of NAMI (formerly National Alliance for the Mentally Ill). Many chapters have referral lists of doctors and therapists who work well with people with a severe mental illness.

- Contact people you know who work in the field of mental health and ask for a referral. If you don't know such a person, or anyone who knows such a person, turn to someone who works in a related health-care field. Think of any nurses, doctors in other specialties, social workers, counselors, or the like that you or any friends or relatives know and could contact.

The most important consideration in choosing a therapist is that the therapist have experience with *the specific kind of illness with which your relative is suffering.* There are many fine psychiatrists, psychologists, and psychotherapists who have no more familiarity with schizophrenia than they do with treating a person with diabetes. You must ask prospective therapists if they have worked with people who have your relative's condition, and if so, how extensively. If finances necessitate that your relative go to a clinic, your options may be limited, but do the best you can to let people know what his or her situation is.

The next most important consideration is your relative's feelings about the therapist. It is crucial that the consumer feel reasonably comfortable with and trusting of the therapist. Very little is likely to be accomplished without a good rapport between them. Patients are far more inclined to take advice from and listen to a doctor or therapist they trust than one they see as incompetent or uncaring.

The therapist should also have realistic expectations for your relative, given the type and severity of the disorder at hand. You don't want a therapist who will expect too much or too little. When expectations are too high, patients experience failure and become discouraged. They will then stop trying to do as much as they can for themselves. On the other hand, if too little is expected, people may become lazy and not live up to their full potential, however limited that may be.

Ideally the therapist will also have a positive, collaborative attitude toward the family. This is becoming more common, though it is still not always possible to find such a therapist. If you have many options, try to find someone who is willing to communicate with you periodically.

If your relative is fortunate enough to find someone with whom she or he feels comfortable and who has experience working with people with a serious mental illness, support the relationship and encourage your relative to stay with that therapist as long as possible. Change is not easy for people with a mental illness, and changing therapists can be particularly upsetting. Even if the therapy is disappointing to you because your relative has not progressed as quickly as you would like, it is advisable that you discourage your relative from switching therapists. The chances of finding someone better are not very high, and you run the risk of having your relative decide to discontinue therapy altogether. This is not to say that a switch should never happen—just that it should be a decision not taken lightly or made frequently.

In selecting a rehabilitation program with your relative, you or the people in charge of making the placement ought to consider the following:

- The person's safety must be ensured. Make sure the facility has the necessary controls to provide for your relative's basic well-being, especially when he or she is suicidal, self-destructive, or potentially violent. Some people need to be in locked facilities, which offer a large degree of supervision.

- The program should, as much as possible, match the level of functioning of your relative. (Ideally, if we had enough funding, there would be a range of programs set up with increasing levels of expectations and responsibility for people; patients would move from one program to another as their level of functioning changed.) Look for programs in which people are allowed as much freedom and responsibility as they can handle. Keep in mind that your relative is not always the best gauge of this. When the residents at the residential facility I ran for years entered the program, many of them said they were not as sick as everyone else there. Over time, as they began to feel more comfortable with the program and the other residents, it became clear that they had more in common with the others than they could first acknowledge.

- Ideally, your relative should also fit in with the patient population. Programs vary in the type of people they serve in general and in who happens to be there at any particular time. This is especially true in smaller residential programs. The level of responsibility in the local six-bed group home may be perfect for your fifty-year-old sister with a bipolar disorder. If, however, it is currently occupied by five eighteen-year-old men with schizophrenia, your sister may not be very comfortable there.

Unfortunately, there are a number of logistical considerations that can influence where your relative goes. Bed availability is a big one in this era of limited services. Your relative may wind up in a program that is not entirely suited to him or her because it is the only one that has an opening when he or she is ready to leave the hospital. A longer stay in the hospital may be an even less desirable option.

Families sometimes fear that if they rely on the mental-health system to care for their relative, he or she will end up in a locked facility and be forgotten. This is not very likely to happen. The more highly supervised or secure a program is, the more it costs to run. Public programs cannot afford to have a patient in a more expensive facility if there is a more appropriate, less expensive bed available. The more freedom and responsibility a program allows its clients, the less expensive a service it is. Thus public service systems are likely to place patients in programs that allow as much freedom and responsibility as possible. This is one instance in which the interests of the patient happen to coincide with prevailing economic interests.

THE PROGNOSIS FOR MENTAL ILLNESS

The long-term picture for people who have a serious mental illness, especially those with schizophrenia, has improved significantly in the last decade. Previously, most professionals in the field held a rather pessimistic view. Their belief was referred to as the rule of thirds. The notion was that about a third of the people with schizophrenia was likely to significantly improve, though still have a somewhat limited life. Another third would remain more seriously disabled by their illness, while the final third would always be so severely disabled as to need almost constant custodial care. Some professionals who adhere to a more traditional medical model of treatment continue to take this view.

There is, however, reason to believe that this view may

create a self-fulfilling prophecy. When people are put in institutions, stripped of all responsibility for their lives, and are told and treated as though they have a chronic, lifelong, disabling illness which will prevent them from accomplishing anything, they begin to believe it. Consequently, they do nothing with their lives and let aides, nurses, and doctors make all their decisions and "take care" of them.

With the development of the consumer movement, described in more detail in the section entitled "Recovery from Mental Illness," and with the new medications now available and changes in the service system, there is reason for a much more optimistic view. There have been studies done in the United States, as well as in Asia and Europe, which suggest the possibility that between fifty to sixty-eight percent of people with schizophrenia can recover or significantly improve. They may have no symptoms or a significant reduction in symptoms, be able to work, and adjust to living in the community.

In recent years, increasing numbers of consumers are taking charge of their lives and treatment with impressive results. They are able to develop new meaning and purpose in life as they grow beyond the catastrophe of mental illness. We are finding that far more positive results occur when people are cared for in a community with a services system that offers individualized treatment planning, supported housing and jobs, early intervention with newer medication, cognitive therapies, and psychosocial rehabilitation programs that teach people how to cope with symptoms and help people learn or relearn social skills and independent living skills. Crucial to people learning to cope effectively with mental illness is having others who believe in them and have hope and confidence that they can live productive lives. Many people are then able to work, have meaningful relationships, and live more independently.

It is difficult to know now, what is possible for the future of people with serious mental illnesses. If we are able to eliminate the stigma of mental illness, and individuals are able to acknowledge that they have an illness and utilize the services and treatments listed above, we are likely to see far better outcomes than we ever have. No one knows how well people with mental illnesses will be able to do in a more supportive environment with ever-improving medications and services.

Of course, not everyone with schizophrenia is currently able to reconstruct such satisfying lives for themselves, and we do not have an entirely supportive and stigma-free society. There continue to be many people whose lives are devastated by the symptoms of mental illness and for whom even the newer medications are ineffective. In many areas the needed services are not available. There are people who have a more severe case or are not able to understand that they have an illness and thus refuse all treatment and services. Approximately ten percent of people with schizophrenia kill themselves, some intentionally, others accidentally.

For reasons that no one fully understands, about fifty percent of people who suffer from schizophrenia get somewhat better when they reach their forties. These are more often males. While the symptoms may not disappear, they do lessen enough for the individuals to experience noticeable relief.

About eighty percent of people with bipolar disorder take medication and are able to do almost all that they would like to do in life. The lives of the other twenty percent are more disrupted by their illness. For them, medication and the other treatments and services mentioned above provide only partial relief from their symptoms. The quality of their lives is more compromised by the illness.

Although there is no sure way to know how severe an illness any individual will have, the following circumstances suggest the possibility of a less severe or less disabling case.

- Early intervention with medication.
- People who have functioned well before they were ill will probably be less disabled by the illness. The areas of functioning to consider include school, work, personal relationships, and interests and skills.
- The absence of a co-occuring serious substance-use disorder.
- An illness that begins later in life may be less severe. Schizophrenia most commonly begins in late adolescence or early adulthood. For males it usually starts between the ages of seventeen and twenty-three, for females, between twenty and twenty-five. While bipolar disorder can appear at any age, it also is likely to be more severe if it appears as early as adolescence or early adulthood.
- The prognosis is usually better if the symptoms begin suddenly, seemingly in response to a specific stressful event. Examples include someone becoming ill after the death of a close relative or after graduating from college. The illness is likely to be more severe when the symptoms begin gradually, over a long period of time, for no apparent reason.
- No family history of severe mental illness suggests the possibility of a less severe case.
- An involved, supportive family improves the ill person's quality of life.
- The absence of symptoms that lead to dangerous or antisocial behavior suggest a better prognosis. If someone hears voices demanding that he or she run down the street naked or jump out of a second story-window, that person will probably need to be in a locked facility, unable to participate in many everyday activities.

- Insight into having a mental illness and accepting the need for treatment.

It is important to remember that none of these is a guarantee. Your relative may first show symptoms of schizophrenia at the age of thirty after getting fired from a good job, and even with a loving family and no known relatives with the illness, still develop a severe case. However, this kind of scenario is not nearly as common as that of the boy who slowly begins to do strange things in high school, increasingly withdraws into his own world, has a mother who is also ill, and continues to gradually deteriorate over time.

Schizophrenia and major affective disorders can be very serious and disabling illnesses. Ultimately families must do their best to make peace with whatever limitations the illnesses impose upon the lives of their loved ones. At the same time families must learn to enjoy whatever good times their ill relative has, appreciate the abilities that remain intact, and try to feel good about any small steps the ill person takes in a positive direction.

3

Essential Skills for Getting Along with People with Mental Illness

THIS CHAPTER FOCUSES ON several key issues for people who interact with someone who has a mental illness. First, the most effective approaches to day-to-day contact with people with a mental illness are described. Then guidelines are presented that can help you in determining what you can realistically expect of your relative and in setting up a structure that fosters his or her well-being. Finally, I present techniques to facilitate communication with someone with a mental illness.

Such skills are useful for everyone who has contact with a person with a mental illness, but are especially important for those who have a relative with a mental illness living at home. Here the need for knowledge increases considerably, and the very quality of life for you and your family is at stake. Having a person with a mental illness living at home is an enormous strain. If poorly handled, the situation can easily wreak havoc on your home and family. You must prepare yourself well by learning and practicing the skills presented here and in the next four chapters.

GENERAL GUIDELINES FOR DAILY LIVING

Respect the Person

Perhaps the most important thing to remember when dealing with people who have a mental illness is that their self-esteem may be extremely low. Their internal worlds may be full of chaos and disorganization, so they may be unable to do many of the things others usually do. Society often reinforces the messages that they are sick, bad, and to be feared. Consequently, they often lack the self-confidence and self-respect necessary to feel good about themselves.

It is therefore vital to treat people with mental illness with *respect*. It is easy to forget that they are doing their best to handle their torturous symptoms. You must always try to find a way to be respectful and to acknowledge their adulthood, even when you need to ask them such things as whether they remembered to brush their teeth, or assure them that you didn't scratch your arm because of what they just thought. Speaking to such people in a condescending manner or infantilizing them will make them feel worse and strain your relationship.

Be Calm and Straightforward

Remain calm, clear, and direct when speaking. Remember that your relative may be hearing strange voices, seeing bizarre things, having racing thoughts, or feeling a mixture of emotions. A long-winded, emotional tirade will likely get lost in the confusion. Short sentences, calmly spoken, have the best chance of being understood. If you are angry about a specific behavior and express this in an emotional way, the ill person will likely not hear or remember any of what you are saying. Thus, the chances are high that he or she will repeat the very behavior that angered you in the first place.

Take Breaks and Pace Yourself

Separating yourself from your ill relative when either of you are particularly upset is also useful. Little is likely to get resolved in the heat of the moment, and your relationship could easily sustain substantial injuries when he or she is most psychotic or upset. If a person or property is in danger, you need to take precautions. If the situation is less severe than that, you would probably do well to take time apart, and suggest that the discussion continue when everyone is feeling better.

The idea of spending minimal amounts of time with someone who is ill when he or she is hurting most is alien to many people. Mental illnesses are, however, different from physical ones in this respect. In the midst of a psychotic episode, people do not always know or remember what they are doing, saying, thinking, and feeling. The presence of family and friends can be more harmful to the relationship than it is helpful to the person. This is especially true if the ill person abuses drugs or alcohol or becomes angry and abusive during an acute episode. Your feelings may be very hurt, and the ill person may wind up feeling guilt afterward, whether or not that person remembers what he or she did.

Keep the long-term picture in mind. You can offer a kind of love, support, and ongoing relationship that no one else can. Your relative will need you in his or her life for many years, through many ups and downs. You will be able to provide this support only if you protect your own health and your relationship with the person. At times this may mean withdrawing from the relationship, taking a break, recognizing that you are tired, or accepting that you are just not able to continue when the illness or substance abuse becomes more severe. Most people with mental illness understand the need to create distance, and often wish they could do the same. They may actually feel worse about their own behavior than about the fact that you have withdrawn from them.

It may take years for you to reach the point of being able to truly accept that your loved one has a mental illness. But until you can accept this, you will not be able to be supportive of your ill relative in the way that he or she needs. If you keep trying to get the person to snap out of it, or attempt to make the symptoms just go away, everyone will wind up frustrated and disappointed.

You have to do everything possible to prevent the unpredictability of the symptoms from wreaking havoc in your life. The illness inevitably takes an enormous toll on everyone. However, it is crucial to prevent your life from becoming as disorganized and chaotic as the life of the ill person. This involves, among other things, figuring out what your limits are, keeping active, and participating in activities that do not include the ill person. Indeed, if your life is less chaotic, it will ultimately be as much of a relief to the ill person as it is to you.

Separate the Person from the Illness

Mental illnesses seriously affect how people think and feel, how they behave, and what they can do. But it is vital for those of us who know and love people who have a mental illness to remember that they are not just "the mentally ill." People with these illnesses are still *people*. They have feelings; they can be easily hurt; their individuality can easily get lost.

They need people in their lives who love and understand them. Many people simply label them as mentally ill, unaware of how much they may have to offer. Friends and family must balance this tendency by remembering to separate the person from the illness.

Learning about symptoms allows you to attribute the symptoms to the illness, not to the person. You must not think of your mother with a bipolar disorder as just an angry, manipulative, hateful person who intends to wreak havoc in your life. She is a victim, and she would probably like nothing more than to be able to think clearly and act normally. You would do far better to hate the illness than to penalize her further for having had the misfortune of being afflicted with it. Many relatives of people with mental illness are able to begin to love their ill relative again once they start hating the symptoms (which include some exasperating behavior) and the illness.

Admittedly, it is difficult not to take particular symptoms personally. Irrational ideas, behavior, and feelings often spill out on whoever is present. It can be useful to think of the situation as similar to that of an infant who has a stomach virus and regurgitates on whoever is holding her. In this case, you would not think of the baby as bad or spiteful. In the same way, think of irrational anger, confused ideas, the inability to plan ahead, and all other symptoms of a mental illness as nothing more than what they are: symptoms. If your relative was in the hospital he or she would likely be directing the symptoms toward the attending nurses or doctors rather than you. For example, the person might be angry at the nurses, thinking they, rather than you, were trying to poison the coffee. The fact that delusions or hallucinations may focus on you means little or nothing about you or your relationship with the ill person.

What can help improve the quality of life and the self-esteem of people with mental illness is your conveying to them that you know that they are ill, that you still love them, and that you want them to be part of your family. We will explore how to include these people in family activities in chapter 7; for now, simply remember that they need to feel a part of some community of people. Many former friends and school-mates grow away from them. Family members are often the only ones who stay with them in the long run.

Your love cannot be based solely on who they used to be or on the hope that they will someday be well. They need to feel that you love them today and that you recognize that they are sick today. We all hope that someday better treat-ments and even a cure will be found. In the meantime we must accept that some people suffer from symptoms that are largely beyond their control. If *you* are able to love and ac-cept them as ill, they will more likely be able to accept their illness and limitations.

Maintain a Positive Attitude

The next most helpful approach, and one that is quite dif-ficult, is keeping a positive attitude. Avoiding feelings of neg-ativity can be a challenge in the face of a seriously disabling illness. Nonetheless, your support and positive outlook will allow people with a mental illness to thrive to the greatest ex-tent possible. People with mental illness may have little to be proud of in their lives. Many of their same-age friends and relatives have gone on to accomplish things that the ill per-sons might never be able to do. You must learn to recognize and comment on any small signs of progress or improvement that you see without being condescending or belittling. Show-ing interest in what your ill relative is doing is more respect-ful than merely noting that he or she is doing something for the first time in a month.

People who have such a difficult time functioning in life,

and who are so misunderstood, need a great deal of praise from those who do understand them. Things in life that the rest of us take for granted can be monumentally difficult for people with a mental illness. Such people may need to be acknowledged, in a way that does not speak down to them, for such things as getting up in the morning, taking care of their personal hygiene, or getting to and from an appointment by themselves.

Keep in mind that one symptom of mental illness is not being able to remember the positive. You can counteract this by repeatedly emphasizing recent achievements. Remind ill people that they are good, strong, and courageous to be able to continue trying to make their lives better. Acknowledge their perseverance. Their lives are far more painful and confusing than most; on some level they may know this, but on another level they can easily sink into feeling bad about themselves for being ill or not being able to do more. You can help them see their struggles from another perspective.

Particularly during bad times, your faith, hopefulness, and encouragement are needed. Even during a crisis you need to try to find some small sign of progress. For example, if your daughter winds up in the hospital for the third time, you could focus on the exasperation, disappointment, and despair that you and she feel. However, it is more useful to acknowledge how hard it must be for her to be back in the hospital and to tell her that you are proud of the fact that this time, for the first time, she saw the episode coming and got to the hospital on her own.

Positive feedback is useful for several reasons. It acknowledges that progress is occurring, even if at a slow pace. It gives your relative something to feel good about at a time when he or she probably has little to feel good about. It lets the person know that you are on his or her side. Also, it will likely help you to keep things in perspective.

People with a mental illness need to feel that, although they may have relapses or may not be able to do certain things in life, they are still worthy of respect and dignity.

DETERMINING REALISTIC GOALS AND EXPECTATIONS FOR YOUR RELATIVE WITH A MENTAL ILLNESS

Discuss goals with your ill relative. His or her interests and wishes are essential to any plans that are developed.

Assess the current overall level of functioning by evaluating the following major areas:

1. *basic skills for independent living:* the ability to shop, cook, clean, manage money, use public transportation. How independently has your relative lived?

2. *interpersonal skills:* the ability to establish and maintain relationships, carry on conversations, and make eye contact.

3. *educational and vocational skills.* Has your relative completed high school or held a job? What type of job and for how long?

A higher-functioning person will:

- be competent in at least two of the above areas
- have no symptoms that consistently interfere with functioning
- show motivation and initiative to progress to a high level of functioning

Establish realistic short-term goals:

Thus, when you show respect for your relative with mental illness, it goes a long way toward balancing the stigma and disrespect to which they are so often subjected.

1. Assess the most recent level of functioning in each major area listed above.

2. Determine in which areas the person is willing and able to improve.

3. Develop small steps toward improvement in one or two of these areas.

4. Choose one area to focus on, and do not move to another until the first has been mastered or the ill person has become too frustrated to continue.

Establish realistic long-term goals: Consider overall past level of functioning; your relative may not exceed this. Persons may be able to return to their past level of functioning if they are able to function at a high level between acute episodes and if over time their level of functioning has not gradually deteriorated.

Avoid common unrealistic expectations—for example:

- that the recovery will be speedy
- that the person will always return to a past level of functioning
- that the person will never again be hospitalized or have a relapse

Remember that the level of functioning of people with mental illness can change rapidly. You must be prepared to quickly adjust your goals and expectations to the current level of functioning.

This is not to say that people with mental illness do not need criticism. They certainly need to know when they do things that are unacceptable. Exactly how to let them know this will be discussed later in this chapter.

DEVELOPING REALISTIC GOALS WITH YOUR ILL RELATIVE

What your loved one can do will depend on many factors, such as the severity of the symptoms, his or her level of motivation, and his or her previous life experience. Most families need to learn to pare down their hopes and expectations to what can realistically be achieved by their ill relative. Figuring out realistic goals will likely require some professional help, but the Quick Reference Guide, Determining Realistic Goals and Expectations for Your Relative with a Mental Illness, summarizes the factors that are usually considered when an assessment of someone's potential is made.

Everyone needs to have goals, dreams, and hopes for the future. However, these goals must be realistic. Families, friends, and professionals can play a useful role in helping an ill person understand that small steps begin them on their way toward long-term goals.

Of course, the agendas that families have for their ill relatives are often very different from those the ill people have for themselves. The most successful plans bridge the two perspectives. People are much more receptive to suggestions when they feel their own ideas or interests—even the most irrational or unrealistic hopes and dreams—are included as part of the plan.

People who have a mental illness often have rather grandiose dreams and goals. They want to be major-league baseball players, nuclear scientists, famous rock musicians, or presidents of international banks. There is no point in telling them that these things will probably never happen. It is far more effective to join with them. Tell them that you, too, hope that someday they will achieve these long-term goals but that in the meantime, since they just got out of the hospital, it might be best for them to think of the first small step they can take to accomplish their goals.

You might suggest that the scientist-to-be, who sleeps till noon and has not read a book for a year, wake up every day at 11:00 A.M. for a week; the next step might be reading the comics in the Sunday paper. The hopeful athlete who has not been out of the house for a week may be willing to start by watering the front lawn; the second step may be taking a walk around the block. The future bank president may need to start by brushing up on arithmetic or learning how to open a checking account.

Sometimes dreams are based on past abilities and talents that, because of the illness, are no longer present. If your daughter was a track star in high school and wants to get back into shape, walk her to the field and see how she does. Help her create a training schedule that is in line with her present abilities.

Often people shy away from previous strengths because it is painful for them to be reminded of what they can no longer do. It is best for you to follow their lead. If your son used to give piano recitals but no longer wants to play, don't push him. Reminding him, even in an effort to be supportive, will probably hurt. He is as painfully aware as you are that he is no longer performing. If you want to brag about him, talk about things he is doing today that he was not doing last week.

Once you pare down your expectations to what is realistic, you can better see and appreciate accomplishments. You can begin to feel, and inspire your relative to feel, encouraged when small goals are achieved. It is these accomplishments that ultimately add up to the attainment of long-term goals.

ESTABLISHING A LOVING DISTANCE

Some questions often asked regarding goals and expectations are: "How involved should I be?"; "How much should we do to help him achieve a goal?"; "If we do too much, how will she ever learn to do things for herself?"; "His life is already so hard. Why shouldn't I do everything I can to make it easier?"

There are no simple answers, and there is no single truth that applies to all situations. Your answers must be closely related to your evaluation of realistic goals and expectations for your ill relative. Your answers must also be influenced by the variable nature of the illness. Since the symptoms tend to be cyclical, you must be prepared to change with them. This means sometimes doing more for your relative and at other times encouraging the person to do more for himself or herself, depending on how sick the person is.

However, it is useful to keep two general principles in mind: first, let people do as much as they can for themselves; second, try to ensure that they feel your love and support. Finding the balance between these two approaches is a challenge that can be thought of as learning to establish a loving distance. Too often family members get polarized around this issue, some representing one side and some the other. Rather than arguing, the task is to find the appropriate middle ground for your relative given the person's current level of functioning.

In addition to assessing ill persons' general level of functioning, other factors to consider include their willingness to do things for themselves, their general level of maturity, and how old they were when they first became ill. Age is relevant because it often correlates with the level of life skills learned and practiced before the onset of the illness. Consider Jim, a sixteen-year-old still living with his parents and not yet finished with high school. He develops schizophrenia. It will be difficult for Jim to learn how to keep a checking account, find an apartment, make new friends, fill out a job application, or even shop and cook dinner for himself. He will likely need a great deal of help learning to do these things after he becomes ill.

On the other hand, consider Sally, a woman who is married, has children and a career, and develops a bipolar disorder at the age of thirty-seven. She has a much better chance of getting back to doing many of the things she used to be able to do. While it may take time and she may not be able to maintain as stressful a job as she once had, she will have an enormous advantage over Jim.

Sometimes the only way to find out what a person can do is by trial and error. The Quick Reference Guide entitled How Involved Should I Be? provides some guidelines as to whether you are expecting too much or too little. Most people—even those who have a mental illness—want to do as much as they can on their own. Given the choice, they prefer to be as independent and responsible as they can. This is a natural desire that reinforces itself when it has been fulfilled. It leaves most people feeling better about themselves.

Sometimes people's fear of failure inhibits their willingness to try new things. By breaking tasks down into small steps, and by providing positive feedback, you will prepare people to take further steps. If you follow this course of action and yet see no improvement, you may want to seek professional help. The illness could be complicated by other psychiatric conditions that require modifying your approach, or you may need to modify your level of expectations, or the method of presenting tasks to the ill person may need to be changed. Whatever the case, a professional counselor can help you.

It is painful for many family members to watch their relative with a mental illness try to do something and not be able to succeed right away. The inclination is to jump in to help or take care of the ill person. But even people who suffer from a mental disorder need to be given the respect and opportunity to make their own mistakes as they master a new skill. Again, it is a matter of finding that delicate balance of encouraging them to try new things while not setting them up to repeatedly fail.

Lastly, as people age, their willingness to try new things

HOW INVOLVED SHOULD I BE?

Do all you can to protect your relative from any clear and present danger to himself or herself or to others. Contact the police or other emergency services if you believe someone's life is at risk.

Consider how the person is meeting his or her basic needs for food, clothing, and shelter and the quality of his or her life. How much you can do in these areas depends on:

1. your relative's willingness to follow your advice
2. how much leverage you have with the person (usually how much support you are providing)
3. your legal relationship with your relative (whether you are his or her conservator or representative payee). Your ability to protect the person or influence his or her life will probably be uncomfortably limited by law.

diminishes. A middle-aged man with schizophrenia who has been ill for twenty years and has lived in a boarding house for the past ten may not want to try a volunteer job or take a class. He has settled into a routine with which he is reasonably content. This may be the best life currently possible for him. While he doesn't do as much as his family wishes for him, his family may need to accept his life as it is rather than try to get him to change. Remember that you are not fully responsible for the quality of your relative's life.

Your relative may be needing more protection or involvement if:

- He engages in self-destructive behavior.
- She does things that could be dangerous to people or property.
- He breaks the law, even if only in minor ways.
- She refuses to follow agreements or treatment plans.
- He does not meet his basic needs for survival (food, clothing, shelter).
- She has a serious substance-use disorder.

Your relative may be overprotected if:

- She exhibits more immaturity than the illness can account for.
- He looks to you or others to do things for him before trying them himself.
- She consistently backs away from taking any small steps toward increased responsibility and independence.

ESTABLISHING A STABLE STRUCTURE

After love, structure is perhaps the most important element of any successful relationship with, or treatment program for, people with mental illness. Without it, they are left adrift, in a tumultuous sea of confusion. With a supportive structure they can, over time, begin to feel more safe and secure.

Thus, you don't throw a surprise birthday party or be your most spontaneous, flamboyant self when you are around people suffering from mental illness. The chaos and disorganization that characterize their internal worlds require a steadying influence. You cannot make their confusion go away. What you can do is provide an external reality that is as calm, consistent, predictable, and structured as possible. In that way he or she knows what to expect from you and what you expect from him or her.

Many events that the rest of us take for granted, such as a simple exchange of amenities or the predictable delivery of a newspaper, can reassure people with a mental illness that all of life is not as disorganized as they feel it is. Having a simple daily routine that includes taking care of their basic needs— getting themselves up, dressed, bathed, and fed—can be very reassuring and important for people with a mental illness. They often need more help than the rest of us in putting a structure or activity for themselves in place and maintaining it. This is a long-term goal for some, but one that is well worth working on.

Conversely, changes in routine can be more upsetting than you might expect. For example, if a friend who frequently visits leaves town, your relative may feel more anxious and confused than usual. This does not mean that you should never leave town; but you do need to understand how your relative is likely to react before, during, and after you take a trip. You need only be supportive and reassure the person that your leaving does not mean that things are as terrible as he or she may feel they are.

Setting Up Rules and Limits

One important aspect of structure is the presence of rules and expectations. Never make assumptions when setting these; no detail is too small to be made explicit. Whether you are planning a brief visit or you live together, things are likely to go better if you both know just what is to happen. For a visit this may mean mentioning how you expect the ill person to dress (if this is a problem), how much time you will spend together, and what you plan to do. If you are living together it may mean writing down the basic rules of the house and specific chores or expectations you have for him or her each day.

Putting things in writing gives people with mental illness a way to remember things that may seem simple or obvious to others. It can also eliminate arguments over what was said or agreed to.

A list of general rules for behavior is a good starting point. This ought not be too lengthy, though it should include any areas that have been problematic. It may be as simple as this:

House Rules

No violence.

No hitting walls.

No slamming doors.

No radio or television after 11:00 P.M.

Clean up kitchen after preparing food.

No use of drugs or alcohol at home.

Having written contracts or agreements can be especially useful when specific behaviors have been repeatedly problematic. Write down exactly which behaviors are unacceptable and exactly what the consequences will be if these behaviors occur. For example:

I understand that I cannot smoke in bed. If I smoke in bed again I will not be allowed to bring cigarettes into the house for one month.

                       _____

            (signature)   (date)

It is best to have your ill relative write out the contract if he or she is able to do so.

Part of having a clear, structured environment or relationship means that clear consequences follow when rules or contracts are broken. Whenever possible, it is a good idea to establish the consequences in advance, and to consult the ill person when doing so. Do not try to develop consequences in the middle of a crisis.

Try to make the consequences relate to the rule to which it pertains. If a person plays the radio past the curfew, he or she might lose the privilege of using it for two days. If the person does not clean up after himself or herself, you might want to assign an extra cleaning chore. The idea is to make the punishment fit the crime whenever possible.

You may set up one or two serious house rules that, if broken more than once, result in the person's being asked to leave—with a less severe consequence set up for the first violation. Whatever seems reasonable and tolerable is fine. The most important thing is that everyone know what the rules are and what will happen if they are not followed. Be sure that you are serious about following through on the consequences you establish; your credibility will depend on this. The Quick Reference Guide entitled Designing and Setting Limits with the Ill Person summarizes the above discussion.

Note especially that you should feel free to change the plan as experience teaches you more about what you can realistically expect from your relative, given the person's current level of functioning. What your relative is able to do will change with the severity of symptoms. Do not, however, get into the habit of abandoning all the limits you set just because he or she is not able to abide by them at a given time. You want to find a balance. Be flexible enough to negotiate or change your expectations with the fluctuating severity of the symptoms, also establish certain nonnegotiable ground rules. For example, you should never allow yourself or anyone else to be exposed to violence or danger.

Choosing Your Battles

Ultimately, you must choose your battles carefully. There are usually many things about people with mental illness that their families would like to change. But many cannot be changed. Those things that can be changed will often take more time and energy than you would prefer. People who have a mental illness are usually able to work on only one area at a time.

Let us say that your daughter with a bipolar disorder sleeps till noon, does not eat well, smokes too many cigarettes, watches too much television, does not groom herself well, and has no structured activities in her life. Assume you have said nothing about any of these issues for a month, and that you have been getting increasingly angry and frustrated with her.

One day you wake up and decide you have reached your limit. You feel things must change. She is twenty-five years old. You tell her that from now on she must wake up at 7:00 A.M., take a shower by eight, have only five cigarettes a day, smoke only on the patio, watch no more than two hours of television a day, and get a job. She will likely do none of it. Rather, she will feel pressured and incompetent. She will want to run away, go to the hospital, or sleep all day, or she will become agitated— depending on which symptoms she exhibits under stress.

In this kind of situation, you must first prioritize. You and she need to decide which area is most important to deal with, and then consider whether this is an area in which she will be

DESIGNING AND SETTING LIMITS WITH THE ILL PERSON

Establish general rules and limits when you and your relative are calm and clear thinking. It is usually a good idea to discuss only one limit at a time, in the following way.

1. Clarify exactly which behavior needs to change, and be realistic about the amount of energy it will take to achieve this.

2. Choose a consequence appropriate to the seriousness of the behavior, and make sure you are prepared to carry it out (for example, you would not want to tell your relative that you will never talk to him or her again if he or she curses in your house). One common consequence is the docking of privileges (money, TV viewing time). Alternately, use rewards to effect a desired change in behav-

willing to do some work. Evaluate with her what changes are possible and determine a realistic time frame. Ideally, you might sit down together and decide that the lack of structure in her life is the most serious problem. The two of you might agree (or, if she is living in your house, you could require) that within a month she will find some activities in which to participate for a minimum of five hours per week. You might help her make a list of the options that interest her, such as participating in a day treatment program, doing volunteer work, taking a class at the local junior college, or finding a part-time job. You might then help her figure out a realistic schedule for exploring whichever options most appeal to her.

ior (dinner out at restaurant of choice, participating in a special outing, and so forth).

3. Make sure your relative understands the rule and its consequence. Don't get defensive or give long explanations. Give your relative a chance to ask questions and give input. Negotiate if this seems reasonable. Putting agreements and contracts in writing is useful.

4. Implement the consequence if necessary. It is essential to follow through in exactly the way you said you would. This, too, is best done when you are calm and clear. Alternately, it is important to acknowledge and praise any aspect of the limit that is observed and to provide any agreed-upon reward.

5. Modify or revise the rule as needed. If a consequence or contract seems inappropriate, change it in a clear and explicit way.

If you are dealing with someone who is less functional, you may decide that the priority is for that person to begin waking up earlier. You can then establish that he or she will get up at, say, 11:00 A.M. each day for the next week. You can determine how this will be accomplished—an alarm clock, a wake-up call. You may then discuss what the reward will be if he or she accomplishes this or what the consequence of nonaccomplishment will be. The Quick Reference Guide entitled Improving Grooming offers an example of how to decide which battles are worth taking on.

IMPROVING GROOMING

People with a mental illness may groom themselves too little or too much, or they may groom themselves in a bizarre manner. Each behavior can be associated with a primary or secondary symptom of a mental illness such as impaired judgment, lack of motivation, obsessive-compulsive behavior, poor reality testing, or self-neglect stemming from low self-esteem. Addressing the behavior may be quite difficult.

To assess whether you want to try to effect a change in a behavior, take a look at the following list and consider which of the categories the behavior falls under (from the most serious to the least).

1. hazardous to the health
2. disruptive or expensive
3. physically offensive

DEVELOPING GOOD COMMUNICATION SKILLS

Studies have shown that families who learn good communication skills can significantly reduce the amount of time their ill relative is likely to spend in the hospital. Experience shows that these skills can also significantly reduce the amount of frustration and stress families have to endure. The more you understand about how people with mental illness think and process information, the more effectively you will be able to communicate with them.

4. inappropriate
5. unattractive or annoying

How much time and energy to devote to the behavior should also depend on how many other problem areas there are, and how serious each of these is. Strategies that have worked to effect change in areas such as grooming are:

1. establishing a specific plan (shower daily, do laundry weekly); setting firm limits with specific consequences and rewards

2. drawing up a written (or verbal) contract with your relative

3. discussion and reasoning

Change will most likely occur slowly, in small steps, when very specific and explicit expectations are consistently made clear.

COMMUNICATING WITH A PERSON
WITH A MENTAL ILLNESS

People who have a mental illness have symptoms and characteristics that require adaptations in the way you communicate to increase your chances of being understood. The following table shows symptoms of mental illness and corresponding adaptations.

Symptom or characteristic	Adaptation
Confusion about what is real	Be simple and straightforward.
Difficulty in concentrating	Be brief; repeat.
Overstimulation	Limit input; don't force discussion.
Poor judgment	Don't expect rational discussion.
Preoccupation with internal world	Get attention first.
Agitation	Recognize agitation and allow the person an exit.
Fluctuating emotions	Don't take words or actions personally.
Fluctuating plans	Stick to one plan.
Little empathy for others	Recognize as a symptom.
Withdrawal	Initiate conversation.
Belief in delusions	Don't argue.
Fear	Stay calm.
Insecurity	Be loving and accepting.
Low self-esteem	Stay positive and respectful.

You can learn specific techniques for talking to your relative that will dramatically increase not only that person's ability to understand you but also your ability to get the results you want when you interact with him or her. The Quick Reference Guide, Communicating with a Person with a Mental Illness, provides some general guidelines to keep in mind whenever you are talking to someone who has a mental illness.

Although we have touched on some of these principles earlier, they warrant emphasis here. The most important guideline is to keep what you say clear and simple. Never forget how much confusion is probably going on inside the ill person. You have the best chance of being heard and understood if you are brief and to the point. A person with a mental illness will often not be able to follow long explanations or complicated, multistep instructions. For example, if you ask your relative (1) to go to the store when he or she has a chance and get enough milk and eggs for the weekend, (2) not to forget to put on a jacket, (3) to close the back door on the way out, (4) to take an umbrella in case it starts raining, and so on, you will only confuse the person. You will get better results if you ask your relative to go to Joe's Market within the next hour and buy a dozen eggs and a half gallon of milk. Then check to make sure he or she is clear about the task and that he or she has enough money to do it.

Also, people who have a mental illness often take what is said quite literally. They may misinterpret jokes and indirect phrasing. If you ask your daughter with a bipolar disorder, for instance, "Do you think you could make your bed?" her response could easily be: "I don't think about my bed at all. I have more important things to think about." Or "Of course I could make my bed. Do you think I'm completely incompetent?" Not having understood your intent, she may walk away feeling hurt and angry, without making her bed. "Please make

your bed" is likely to be a much more effective way of word-
ing your request.

Timing is of the essence. You must carefully choose when
to say things to people with mental illness. If they are particularly upset, preoccupied with their internal voices, or beset
with other symptoms, you would be wise to postpone bringing up a serious or difficult issue, such as goals. If possible,
wait until they are as calm and clear thinking as they can
be. This does not mean you ought to wait weeks, only that
you would do well to pay attention to their emotional state if
you want to have a serious conversation or exchange. Letting
people know that you have something you need to talk to
them about, and then allowing them to be involved in deciding when the discussion will happen will often get you more
cooperation.

People who have mental illness are often unable to clearly
communicate what they need or what upsets them. They may
not even be consciously aware of such things. Often it is more
important to pay attention to their behavior and emotional
state than to what they say. For example, you have a daughter who has schizophrenia. You tell her that to live with you
she must follow certain rules, and although she tells you she
thinks that is ridiculous, she nonetheless follows the rules.
When you tell her that you are going on a vacation, she says
she thinks that is great, but then becomes depressed or angry.

Small improvements in communication will make noticeable differences. However, while good communication often
makes things better, it will not solve all problems or make
you relative well.

Making Positive Requests

Making a request of someone who has a mental illness
seems, at first glance, like a simple process. There are, however,

certain aspects of the process that can determine whether your request will be heard the way you intended it to be. These are outlined in the Quick Reference Guide entitled Making Positive Requests.

Requests are different from demands. Demands threaten people and make them angry, defensive, and negative. Requests are also different from wishes, hopes, or expectations that another person will do or say what you would like; these are generally unstated and often result in frustration because the other person does not know what you would like. Making positive requests in a direct, pleasant, and honest way helps you to get what you want and need from others. Remember that people who have a severe mental illness tend to be especially sensitive to the emotional climate of others who are in their presence. You must therefore pay particular attention to your manner, expression, and body language if you want the person to correctly understand what it is you want to communicate.

For example, let's say you want your sister with bipolar disorder to help you mow the lawn. If when you talk to her you look angry, sound cold and distant, or begin with a list of her shortcomings or your irritation with how little she does for you, she may shy away from wanting to do anything with you. She may feel hurt and confused, without being able to articulate why. If your tone is demanding or nagging, she may become angry and defensive. If, on the other hand, you say, "I would really appreciate it if you would help me mow the lawn," you have a reasonably good chance of being well received. It works well to say how you will feel if the ill person does what you are asking.

Phrasing things in this way often takes quite a bit of practice. If you are unaccustomed to doing so, you can expect to slip back into old habits occasionally as you learn new ones. Of course, the more you practice, the better you will become. Since communicating in this way usually produces such good results, reinforcement for continuing to make the effort is built-in.

Expressing Negative Feelings

Negative feelings such as anger, annoyance, irritation, hurt, frustration, uptightness, anxiety, uneasiness, fear, sadness, and unhappiness occur as part of coping with the problems of life. When negative feelings are expressed directly and clearly, they can be a constructive force in a healthy family— one that solves its problems without letting them fester. Ex-

---

MAKING POSITIVE REQUESTS

To make a *positive request*:

1. Look at and lean toward the other person.
2. Have a pleasant facial expression or smile when you start to speak.
3. Use a warm tone and accentuate positive feelings.
4. Specify and clarify exactly what you would like the other person to do or say. For example: "Mowing the front lawn would be a big help to me." "It would be a terrific load off my mind if you would take your medication each morning." "It's important to me that you see your doctor."
5. Let the person know how you would feel if your request was granted. Accent positive feelings.

pressing negative emotions in constructive ways allows family relationships to be strengthened rather than weakened.

Most people have difficulty in finding a calm, clear, effective way of expressing negative feelings. Nevertheless, it is important that you develop a way to let your ill relative know that you are upset about something that he or she has or has not done. It is important to pay attention to how and when you do this. The general principles for making a positive request or statement apply here, too, and are outlined in the Quick Reference Guide entitled Expressing Negative Feelings Directly.

For example:

"I would feel much better if you would
_____."
"I would really appreciate it if you would
_____."
"It would make me feel good if you would
_____."

Topics that might be dealt with using positive requests include asking the ill person to:

- take medication regularly
- engage in a particular activity
- do a favor
- engage in conversation
- provide some help in solving a problem

Match your tone and body posture to the content of what you are saying. If you are smiling or reading a newspaper when you tell your brother that you are angry that he did not clean up after himself, he will probably not take you seriously. At all costs, avoid stockpiling resentments until some

EXPRESSING NEGATIVE FEELINGS DIRECTLY

To express negative feelings directly:

1. Express yourself when the problem behavior occurs. Don't wait until later (unless it is impossible to be reasonably calm and clear at the moment).

2. State specifically what it is that the other person has done or said (or failed to do or say) that is producing the negative feeling in you. Be clear and specific. For example: *"When you pace back and forth and then spend so much time just standing and staring into space . . ."*

3. Tell the other person how his or her behavior is affecting you by stating the feeling you are experiencing. Be direct and honest. For example: "When you pace back and forth and then just stand and stare into space, *I feel very sad. I feel uneasy, and it's hard for me to stay in the house and watch you.*"

4. Request that the person change his or her behavior or ask the person to help you solve the problem by coming up with an alternative solution. For example: "When you pace back and forth and

little thing causes you to explode with an arsenal of verbal assaults.

Also, do not launch into a generalized character attack, such as telling your brother that he is a lazy slob. Instead, gently but firmly say that when he doesn't clean up his dishes,

then stand and stare into space, I feel sad and uneasy. *I would feel much better if you would try to do something constructive and helpful in the house. Can you think of some things that you could do right now?"* Other possibilities:

"It really hurts my feelings when you _____. Please stop."

"When you don't _____, I feel uncomfortable. I would feel much better if you would do it."

"I get so frustrated and irritated when you _____. I'd appreciate your helping me by _____."

5. Look at the other person when you are expressing negative feelings. This adds impact to what you are saying.

6. Lean toward the person or come close to him when you are expressing negative feelings. This helps to make the expression more direct and helps the person hear you correctly.

7. Have a serious expression on your face, in tune with your feelings and message.

8. Use a firm tone of voice consistent with the feelings you are expressing.

GUIDELINES FOR DEALING WITH A PERSON WITH A MENTAL ILLNESS

- Be respectful: talk to adults as adults.
- Be calm, clear, and direct in communication.
- Be as consistent and predictable as you can.
- Set clear limits, rules, and expectations.
- Keep a loving distance.
- Accept the person as ill.
- Attribute the symptoms to the illness.
- Don't take the symptoms or the illness personally.
- Reduce contact when your relative is especially ill.
- Maintain a positive attitude, even during failures.
- Allow the ill person to be unable to do things yet retain dignity.

you feel angry. Then go on to tell him exactly what you would like done differently in the future. The more specific you can be, the better. For example, "After you make yourself a sandwich, I would feel better if you would put everything away and wipe off the counter."

This method of communication has made a significant difference for many people. Remember to include the three main elements: exactly what the person did, how you felt about it, and how you would like him or her to behave in the future. Make sure your tone and facial expression are consistent with what you are saying. The sooner you can discuss the problem the better; wait only long enough to organize your thoughts and to be able to present yourself calmly and clearly.

- Notice and praise any positive steps or behavior.
- Offer frequent praise and, separately, specific criticism.
- Focus on current functioning and achieving the best life possible in the present.
- Translate long-term goals into a series of short-term goals.
- Help the ill person attain realistic short-term goals.
- Take an *I don't know* attitude in response to long-term questions.
- Don't let the illness create total chaos in your life.
- Be active; engage in activities without the ill person.
- Continue to educate yourself and talk to supportive people.

THE RULES REVISITED

The Quick Reference Guide entitled Guidelines for Dealing with a Person with a Mental Illness gives twenty rules that will help you make your interactions with your ill relative more satisfying.

To some extent you will need to apply these guidelines selectively. The only way to know for sure what works best with any one individual or family is through trial and error.

SPOUSES

Issues that spouses and partners of people with mental illness face have some similarities with and some differences from those of parents, adult children, and siblings. As a group, spouses have tended to get less support and feel less connected to each other and to family members than do other relatives. This is unfortunate, as their needs, problems, and pain are just as intense as anyone who loves a disabled person. Spouses, like others, must find a way to cope with the grief, stigma, stress, and confusion that mental illness brings. They face additional financial and social problems. They need to educate themselves about the illness and treatments, and to learn to separate the person from the illness. They will be better able to cope if they can find a way to understand symptoms and noncompliance with treatment, without taking it personally or seeing it as a lack of caring or a betrayal. Spouses must try to find the support and nurturance they need, as well as ways to take breaks from the person and seek relief from the additional stress they are under.

Among the most difficult issues facing partners is whether or not to continue with the relationship. Many people decide they are not able to endure persistent symptoms or cannot live with someone who is unable to sustain the kind of relationship they originally envisioned and want for themselves. This is an extremely difficult decision to make. Partners often feel very torn and guilty just thinking about leaving someone who is ill and in need of care. They may love the person, care deeply about him or her, yet decide they are unable or unwilling to make the kind of compromises and accommodations necessary to live with someone who has a disabling illness. People must decide what their limits are and what is tolerable for them. Whatever they decide, it is rarely without a great deal of ambivalence and mixed feelings.

Those who stay, perhaps feeling a need to honor their marriage vows or the commitment they have made, must often significantly alter their lives and expectations for the relationship. They must find ways of coming to terms with living with a partner who periodically needs extensive caretaking, is not always able to return the support and attention they want, and is unable to consistently carry his or her share of responsibilities. They may have to alter their ideas of family roles, such as the father needing to assume primary child-rearing responsibilities, or the wife struggling to accept that her husband at times requires the kind of attention and responses more frequently given to children.

Spouses are often faced with myriad small and large decisions ranging from whether or not to invite company to the house to whether to have children. As with so many issues families face, there are no simple answers. Some people with a mental illness are able to be effective parents while others are not. It certainly adds a very significant level of stress to individuals and relationships. Partners sometimes feel they are a single parent caring for an additional child. Spouses may have to decide whether to assume control over financial matters. These are complicated and difficult choices.

It takes an enormous amount of time, energy, and patience to be in a relationship with someone who experiences repeated acute episodes. Sometimes the period following a hospitalization and return home can be even more stressful than a crisis. When people are acutely ill, partners tend to rally and keep expectations low. Some period of recuperation is usually anticipated when an ill person returns home. It is when the recovery process takes longer and goes more slowly than hoped for that things may become even more difficult. Everyone is drained from all that has occurred and patience can wear thin. The couple may struggle with issues concerning how to reintegrate the ill person into family life. It may not be clear what levels of expectations are realistic. At this time, a spouse may be in as much need of support as the consumer. This fact can be easily overlooked.

Partners must pay particular attention to getting their own needs met at this time. This may be done through contact with supportive friends and family or by seeking professional counseling. During and following acute episodes, relationships are subjected to severe stress and strain. This should lessen over time. If the stress and strain does not appear to be lessening, or if it gets worse, it may be advisable for the couple to seek couples counseling.

Spouses are rarely comfortable being solely in the role of a caretaker for their partner. Most also want to feel that they have a relationship where they can also receive love and support. When love and support are not forthcoming for extended periods of time, it is natural for resentments to build. It will take time for these feelings to subside.

Rebuilding trust is another issue with which couples struggle. Trust can be broken and damage done to a relationship—especially during manic episodes or when substance abuse occurs. Again, much time and patience is often required to repair such damage. Either partner may become angry or frustrated with the length of time it takes to repair the relationship. If such feelings persist, couples are again encouraged to seek professional help from a therapist familiar with the illness.

There are many times when a spouse might want to seek counseling in the course of dealing with a partner's illness. These times include the period shortly after the onset of an illness and following acute episodes (as described above). It is during these periods that spouses are most in need of support and education about mental illness, as well as assistance in making some of the complicated decisions they face. It is not necessary or advisable for a spouse to isolate during these difficult times. Although that sometimes feels like the course of least resistance, it is not the one that is likely to yield the best outcome. Spouses must struggle against the inclination many feel to suffer silently or alone. Feeling overwhelmed with all the decisions and responsibilities they face, it is easy to forget that there are many people dealing with similar situations. Finding others and talking with them can provide enormous comfort and support. Spouses are in particular need of mastering the skills discussed in this and the next three chapters to best cope with all the additional stress in their lives.

4

Handling the Basic Symptoms—Hallucinations, Delusions, and Disorganized Speech—and Minimizing Relapses

*F*RIENDS AND FAMILIES OF people with a mental illness frequently ask questions such as the following: "What do I say when he starts talking about messages he has received from the television?"; "What do I do when she starts to gesture in strange ways?"; "What can I do to prevent my relative from getting sicker and having to go to the hospital again?" These are important questions, and although there is often no way to prevent someone with a serious mental illness from having hallucinations, delusions, or relapses or engaging in bizarre behavior, there are several techniques you can use to make your responses more effective and your interactions more rewarding when you are faced with such situations. There are also things you can do to minimize the frequency with which your relative is likely to have a relapse.

RESPONDING TO DELUSIONS
AND HALLUCINATIONS

There are several principles to keep in mind when you are dealing with people who are delusional or who you suspect are hallucinating. First, while the things they hear, see, smell, feel, or believe may not be observable to you, they are powerfully real to them. These people are genuinely hearing voices or seeing images; they are convinced of their beliefs. You must not dismiss or minimize the impact of these experiences. If you do, you will succeed only in discrediting yourself.

The second principle to remember is that a variety of emotional experiences accompany delusions and hallucinations, ranging from the quite pleasant and entertaining to the terrifying. It is often more important to respond to your relative's emotional state than to the content of the delusional beliefs or hallucinations. For example, let's say your mother is frightened because she believes that the devil will be appearing at nine o'clock to torture her. It is more useful to discuss with her what can be done to help her feel safer than to try to persuade her that the devil will not be arriving at nine.

Lastly, you must take whatever measures are necessary to ensure your own safety, and that of your relative, and to maximize everyone's level of comfort. There is no reason to try to stop a symptom from occurring if your relative is able to go about his or her business without bothering anyone. For example, let's say your relative is able to maintain a part-time volunteer job and has a few friends. When the person comes home in the evening he or she receives messages from the television, but they are not particularly upsetting. In this case, you need not intervene. If, however, *you* feel extremely uncomfortable when your relative talks about what the television voices say, you can request (in the manner described in chapter 3) that he or she refrain from doing so in your presence. Some people will be able to comply with such a request, and some will not.

If, on the other hand, your ill relative is extremely upset by what his or her voices or the television say, you will want to help him or her find a way to feel less upset. How to go about this depends on the individual involved. You may be able to reassure the person that you believe he or she is in no immediate danger, in spite of what he or she is hearing. For example, if a voice is telling your son he is about to be killed, you can tell him that you do not believe that to be true or that you will call the police or do whatever is necessary if anyone tries to harm him. (Keep in mind that your statements may confuse him as well. If, for example, a voice is telling him that his father is about to poison him and his father then tells him that he has nothing to worry about, he may not know whom to believe.)

If your ill relative is angered by the voices or by delusions, you can talk with him or her about what to do to feel less angry. This may be as simple as the person's taking a warm bath, listening to music, or getting together with a friend, or it may mean his or her calling the doctor, taking more medication, or visiting the psychiatric emergency services.

People vary in the degree to which they are convinced that their delusions are true or their hallucinations real. Some people can learn to understand them as a symptom of their illness. They may turn to you for a reality check, and you can then feel free to tell them that you believe the experience is a trick their mind is playing on them, a hallucination, or whatever term best allows them to understand the experience. Other people are completely convinced that the experience is real. They may even think that those who do not believe them are crazy or part of a plot to drive them insane.

What you want to avoid at all costs is arguing about whether the delusions are true or the voices are real: you will never win such an argument. If you are forced to take a stand on this issue, you can respectfully say that you know the experience is true or real for them, and that you happen to have a different experience or opinion.

HANDLING HALLUCINATIONS

Someone may be hallucinating if he or she:

1. talks to himself or herself in a conversational or emotional way, seeming to respond to questions or statements from others (not "Where did I put my keys?"—type comments)
2. laughs, smiles, or frowns for no apparent reason
3. appears distracted or preoccupied; has difficulty staying focused on a conversation or a task
4. appears to be seeing something you can't see

People learn to deal with hallucinations, with practice, by using one or a combination of the following techniques:

1. talking to a therapist or someone else
2. increasing their antipsychotic medication
3. telling the voices to leave them alone
4. ignoring the voices, images, smells, tastes, or sensations
5. focusing on a task or activity
6. listening to loud music (preferably with headphones)
7. stopping the use of alcohol and street drugs which can increase hallucinations

---

People also vary greatly in their sensitivity to the fact that they have delusions or hallucinations. They may have been mocked for their beliefs and experiences, and learned to hide

---

In a supportive, empathetic, calm manner, you can:

1. Ask if the person just heard or saw something and if so, what it was.
2. Get enough information to determine how he or she is feeling about the experience.
3. Discuss ways to deal with the feelings or underlying needs that emerge—what will help him or her feel safe, what he or she can do to feel more in control.
4. Discuss the possibility that the experience is a symptom, a hallucination, or whatever term he or she may use to label it.
5. Remind the person, if necessary, of any relevant limit on his or her behavior, such as not screaming.

You should *not*:

1. Make fun of the person or his or her experience.
2. Act shocked or alarmed by the experience.
3. Tell the person the experience is not real or casually dismiss or minimize it.
4. Enter into lengthy discussions about the content of the hallucination or why someone might be saying the things he or she is hearing.

---

them from others, lie about them, or deny having them. It is therefore not always easy to know if someone is delusional or hallucinating.

With time and experience you can learn to recognize the signs indicating that your relative may be hallucinating or delusional. He or she may stare into space as if watching or hearing something, may talk to himself or herself, or may start laughing for no apparent reason. It is best to give such a person the message that you understand that he or she is having these experiences and that it is okay with you. Let the person know you will not be disturbed or angry—that you want only to help make his or her life as comfortable as possible. Of

RESPONDING TO DELUSIONS

Do not question or discuss the details of delusional statements in any depth. Do not try to convince or argue people out of a delusion. It won't work.

Do not tell people that what they are saying is crazy, delusional, or untrue—*unless* that is specifically asked of you. Even then, do so with caution.

If your relative is calm, listen neutrally, calmly, and respectfully. Then do any or all of the following:

1. Respond to any nondelusional remarks that have been made.
2. Lead the conversation away from the delusional content.
3. Explicitly, but nonjudgmentally, express your desire to change the subject.

course if the hallucinations or delusions lead to behavior that is unacceptable, such as yelling in the middle of the night, you will want to set limits on such behavior.

It often happens that delusions or hallucinations start out being rather benign. People may first hear voices that whisper their name or say funny things. However, over time the voices often become more troublesome. They may begin to berate the people, calling them names or telling them to do things that are dangerous to themselves or to others. Some people learn over time to handle the voices by talking back to them, telling them to leave them alone, or by focusing on an activity. Others can learn to ignore the voices. Some people are

---

If your relative insists on your making a comment about the delusional material, you can:

1. Say you don't know or hedge.
2. Acknowledge the person's reality and, being as respectful of his or her opinion as you are of your own, explain that there is an honest difference of opinion or perception between you.

If strong feelings accompany the delusions, you can:

1. Acknowledge or address the emotions (fear, anger, anxiety, sadness) without commenting on the delusion.
2. Offer assistance in coping with the feelings—for example, you can ask, "What can you or I do to help you feel more safe?"

helped by an increase in antipsychotic medication when these symptoms become more severe. This, of course, should be supervised by a doctor.

The two Quick Reference Guides, Handling Hallucinations and Responding to Delusions, provide handy reminders of what to do if you suddenly find yourself with someone you think may be experiencing one of these psychotic symptoms.

RESPONDING TO DISORGANIZED SPEECH

Principles and techniques similar to those presented in the two preceding Quick Reference Guides apply when you are dealing with someone whose speech becomes extremely disorganized. Just as you don't need to feel bad about the fact that you cannot see someone else's hallucination, you don't need to worry about the fact that you cannot make sense out of some or all of what the person is saying. You need to accept the fact that his or her mind is working in a way that is different from yours. There is no need to be frightened unless the person seems extremely angry, threatening, and out of control. It is best to concentrate on conveying your respect and regard for the person.

Try to find some common ground upon which you can interact. This may mean initiating topics that you think may be of interest, just listening, or playing a game. Sometimes you can pick out one thought in a string of seemingly unrelated ideas and respond to that. It often helps to respond to emotional tone. If your relative seems amused by what he or she is saying, you can comment on the fact that he or she seems to be feeling good and say you are glad to see that. If the person seems frightened, you might ask if he or she is scared and try to help him or her find ways to feel less so.

The most important thing you want to communicate is

that you care. You can do this merely by spending a little time with the person, treating him or her with respect, and paying attention to his or her concerns. Think of it as trying to communicate with someone who speaks a foreign language: you can be warm and convey concern without being able to understand a single word.

How clearly people with a serious mental illness can think and consequently talk will vary greatly from day to day or week to week. Try to enjoy the clearer times with them, and model for them ways of tolerating the confused times. When the confusion becomes more severe and continues for several days, it may indicate the beginning of a relapse, and it would be wise to discuss with your relative and any professionals involved a temporary increase or change in medication.

Your relative may easily get as lost in his or her confusion as you do. He or she may be trying, in spite of it, to make some kind of contact with you. If you can be welcoming of these efforts, your relationship will be all the better for it.

HANDLING ANGER IN SOMEONE
WITH A MENTAL ILLNESS

Friends and relatives are often frightened when their ill relative becomes angry. It is less difficult for most people to learn to deal with irrational fear, sadness, delusions, and hallucinations than with irrational anger. All the myths of the mentally ill as violent psychotic killers come welling up.

However, people with mental illness usually have a much louder bark than bite. The principles discussed above apply here and are equally effective. The only difference is that you need to determine the likelihood of danger or violence. I will deal more extensively with violence in chapter 5, but for now let us focus on managing anger. The Quick Reference Guide,

Handling Your Ill Relative's Anger, summarizes the steps to take. If your relative has never been violent, there is no reason to suspect that he or she will be so now.

The first issue to pay attention to is your own emotional state. If both of you are equally angry and upset, it is best to separate until at least *you* calm down. You will be most ef-

HANDLING YOUR ILL RELATIVE'S ANGER

If you are both angry and fear losing control, it is best to separate, protecting everyone from injury.

If your relative is angry and you are not:

1. Remain as calm as you can; talk slowly and clearly.
2. Stay in control. Either hide your fear, as it may cause the situation to escalate, or tell the person directly his or her anger is frightening you.
3. Do not approach or touch the person without his or her request or permission to do so.
4. Allow the person an avenue of escape.
5. Do not give in to all demands; keep limits and consequences clear.
6. Try to determine whether the anger is completely irrational and thus a symptom of the illness, or if there is a real cause that you can validate.
7. Do not argue irrational ideas.
8. Acknowledge the person's feelings and express your willingness to try to understand what the person is experiencing.

fective in handling the situation if you can present yourself in a calm, clear manner. The communication skills discussed in chapter 3 are especially important when emotions are running high. You want to exude a sense of being in control and on top of the situation. Often a reassuring, calming tone of voice can, in a relatively short time, quiet someone's irra-

9. Help your relative figure out what to do next.

10. Protect yourself and others from injury; some outbursts cannot be prevented or stopped.

If angry outbursts are a recurring problem, wait until everyone is calm and then brainstorm acceptable ways in which the person can handle angry feelings and remain in control. These might include:

1. being clear and direct at the time of minor annoyances so the anger doesn't get bottled up and explode

2. venting some energy via exercise, hitting something safe (a pillow), or yelling in a secluded place

3. leaving the situation or taking some time out to write in a journal or count to oneself

4. taking an additional dose of medication, if prescribed

5. taking an anger-management class

tional anger and fear. Remember that fear and hurt are often what lie beneath an angry exterior.

Pay attention also to your physical presence. You don't want to crowd someone who is upset. One situation that sometimes leads people who have a mental illness to strike out is their feeling cornered or trapped. It is therefore a good idea to leave them easy access to an exit or to position yourself so that you can leave if emotions get too heated. Unless you are sure they will feel comfortable with your physical touch when they are upset, avoid initiating any physical contact.

Acknowledge that they are angry or upset. Be as understanding as you can about the reasons they are upset (if any of those reasons are clear to you). Do not minimize or dismiss the fact that they are having strong feelings. Help them focus on what they need to do to calm down. In fact, you may want to say explicitly that calming down needs to be the first order of business and that the particulars of why they are angry can be dealt with when they feel less upset.

You need to be clear about what sort of behavior is acceptable, even if they are angry. If they are threatening to throw something or are yelling in a way that will disturb neighbors, you must calmly but firmly set a limit. For example, tell them that unless they stop engaging in the behavior, they will have to leave.

If things get to the point that you feel threatened or think physical violence is likely to occur, or if you want someone to leave your home and he or she refuses, you have the option of calling the police. Calling the police when a friend or relative is involved is very upsetting. It is, however, an option that you may have to use at some point with a person who has a serious mental illness. The speed and nature of police response will depend on how serious the police assess the situation to be and how busy they are. In smaller communities the police are often more willing and able to arrive promptly than in larger urban areas, where crime rates are higher. While it is always unpleasant to have the police intervene, it is sometimes the best way to handle a situation and to ensure everyone's safety. The ill person will usually wind up in a place that can provide the external controls he or she needs.

MINIMIZING RELAPSES

By definition schizophrenia, major depression, schizoaffective disorder, and bipolar disorder are cyclical illnesses. The symptoms wax and wane, often for no apparent reason. Accepting this fact can help you feel less guilty and less inclined to tiptoe around your relative out of fear of triggering an episode.

Periods when the symptoms get worse are called *acute episodes* or *relapses*. For someone with a bipolar disorder they are the times when the depression is extreme or the mania occurs. For people with schizophrenia, relapses may consist of an increase in psychotic symptoms or by extreme "negative symptoms" such as withdrawal, passivity, and an inability to provide for basic self-care. Relapses may also be characterized by behaviors that pose a danger to self or others. Relapses often end with multiple visits to emergency psychiatric services or hospitalization.

The truth is, the illness manifests itself somewhat uniquely in each person. Your goal is to learn your relative's patterns. How does he or she act when the symptoms are less severe? How does he or she behave when the symptoms are getting worse? You then need to learn, usually by trial and error, which measures are most effective when your relative becomes more acutely ill.

For example, early warning signs often appear as the symptoms worsen. These tend to be idiosyncratic to each individual, so you must learn what your particular relative does when getting sicker. Do sleep or eating habits change? Does he or she suddenly seem euphoric and spend large amounts of money (which he or she may or may not have)? Is the person

MINIMIZING RELAPSES

Encourage the most therapeutic day-to-day lifestyle, including regular exercise, recreational activities, daily routine, eating a balanced diet, and abstaining from the use of illegal drugs and alcohol.

Identify the early warning signs, such as:

1. any marked change in behavior patterns (eating or sleeping patterns, social habits)
2. absent, excessive, or inappropriate emotions and energy
3. any idiosyncratic behavior that preceded past relapses
4. odd or unusual beliefs, thoughts, or perceptions
5. difficulty in carrying out usual activities
6. impairment in communication

When warning signs appear, do the following, making sure to involve your relative as much as possible:

1. Notify the doctor and request an evaluation for increase in medication.
2. Maintain involvement in any ongoing psychiatric treatment program.

giving away possessions? Is he or she hallucinating more and becoming more agitated? You may even notice, over time, that seemingly routine behaviors, like wearing red clothing or getting a dramatic change in hairstyle, often precede a relapse.

3. Responsibly decrease any known environmental stressors.

4. Minimize (within reason) any changes in routine.

5. Maintain essential aspects of the most therapeutic lifestyle, especially keeping the environment as calm, safe, and predictable as possible.

6. Discuss your observations with your relative and talk about the steps he or she might take to prevent another relapse, hospitalization, or incarceration.

Minimize the impact of a relapse by being prepared:

1. Have a crisis plan ready for yourself.

2. Keep emergency phone numbers and procedures in a convenient place.

3. Know your limits and how you will proceed if they are exceeded.

4. Tell your relative calmly and clearly what your limits are, exactly what they need to do next, and what you will do if those limits are exceeded. For example, "You may not throw things in this house. Please put that cup down immediately. If you throw it, I will call the police."

Although there is enormous variation in patterns, each individual pattern, over time, has a recognizable form. Once you have lived through several relapses you are likely to recognize this pattern. You then want to try to intervene as early as possible. You may not be able to prevent a relapse, but you may be able to help minimize its length and severity. This will be of great value to someone who has gone through a painful psychotic, manic, or major depressive episode. Your objective is to help the person utilize interventions as soon as the signs begin. You might want to urge temporarily minimizing the amount of stress and change that the person has to deal with, increasing medication, or even arrange for a brief hospitalization.

Over time the ill person may learn to recognize the signs that signal the onset of an acute episode. If he or she can do this, the chances of early intervention and a less severe episode increase dramatically. However, many people, especially those who are more severely ill, are never able to do this. The Quick Reference Guide, Minimizing Relapses, outlines what you need to know in order to be prepared for and best handle relapses. The topic is discussed further on pages 241–45.

HELPING THE ILL PERSON MANAGE STRESS

Helping a person with a mental illness learn how to deal with stress is one of the most important things a family or social rehabilitation program can do. Stress alone does not cause symptoms or acute episodes, but lowered stress has been shown to help keep symptoms and relapses to a minimum.

As suggested by the Quick Reference Guide entitled Helping the Ill Person Manage Stress, managing stress can be broken down into three parts. The first is recognizing what causes a particular individual to feel stress. Several examples

HELPING THE ILL PERSON MANAGE STRESS

1. Notice what seems to cause stress in your ill relative. It is important to discuss this in advance with your relative so that you both can prepare yourselves if you know a stressor is about to occur. Common stressors include:
   - major changes in one's routine
   - loss of or separation from loved ones
   - anniversaries, birthdays, and holidays
   - attempting something new and failing
   - attempting something new and succeeding
   - getting involved in an intimate relationship
   - seeing someone close, or with whom the ill person identifies, get sick or become worse

2. Notice possible connections between events (stressors) and feelings (reactions), and discuss such linkages with the ill person.

3. Take note of and discuss (if possible) those things that help the ill person deal with the feelings associated with stress. These may include:
   - minimizing other changes for the time being
   - engaging in hobbies or pastimes that the ill person enjoys and finds reassuring
   - spending time alone
   - talking with a friend, relative, or doctor
   - increasing medication
   - using any relaxation, meditation, or other technique that works for the person
   - exercising

of common stressors are listed, but this list is by no means exhaustive. Remember that stress is idiosyncratic; what is stressful for one individual may not be so for another. Your relative must try to learn what makes him or her feel stress. You need to suspend all judgment about what you think ought or ought not be stressful and accept that he or she will have reactions to things that may seem inconsequential to you.

Many people who have a mental illness have a difficult time understanding that there is a connection between events that happen in their lives and the way they feel or act. It is therefore useful to point out such connections to them. But you must do so gently, with care. And do not expect them to agree immediately; you may have to present your idea numerous times before your relative can accept the possibility that any such connection exists. For example, when talking

---

HOW TO BEHAVE AROUND PEOPLE WHO HAVE A MENTAL ILLNESS

1. Treat them with respect, even if you do not understand some of the things they do or say.
2. Be as supportive, accepting, and positive as you can.
3. Be calm, clear, direct, and brief in your communication with them.
4. Engage them in casual conversation or activities with which you and they are comfortable.
5. Do not touch them or joke with them unless you know them well and know they are comfortable with such interactions.

to your father with schizophrenia, you might say something like, "I notice that for the past three years, around Christmastime, you have become more ill and wound up in the hospital. This seems to be a difficult time of year for you." He may deny the connection. If so, there is nothing more you can say about it at that point; if he winds up in the hospital or feels stressed again next year, you could again present him with the connection. If, on the other hand, he agrees, you can go on to explore what it is about Christmas that is difficult for him and how things can be adjusted to minimize the stress.

Sometimes you may observe a particular behavior that suggests to you that your relative is having a hard time. Is he or she sleeping more than usual, pacing a lot, getting angry more easily, not doing routine activities or chores, or not tak-

6. Do not ask a lot of questions about their lives.

7. Do not give advice unless they request it.

8. Do not discuss in any detail religion, politics, or any other topic that is highly emotional for them, as these topics may be intertwined with delusional thinking. Explain that these are personal or individual issues that you prefer not to discuss.

9. If they behave in ways that are unacceptable to you, calmly tell them *specifically* what they can and cannot do.

ing care of his or her personal hygiene? Once you identify such behaviors, you can suggest to your relative that these indicate that he or she is feeling stress or having difficulty. The person may agree or disagree, but you can at least broach the subject with your new understanding.

The third aspect of helping your relative manage stress is to find things your relative can do that will reduce the amount of stress he or she feels. Perhaps simply talking about what is bothering the person can reduce the stress. Alternately, you might suggest that he or she develop a list of general things to do that help the person feel better when he or she is having a hard time. It might be as simple as drinking a glass of warm milk or taking a bath, or it may involve engaging in an activity or applying relaxation techniques.

TIPS FOR FRIENDS AND RELATIVES

Your friends and relatives may also need pointers on how to act around your ill relative. This information is summarized in the Quick Reference Guide entitled How to Behave Around People Who Have a Mental Illness, and should be familiar to you by now. It may be useful to give your friends a copy of these guidelines.

Managing More Severe Symptoms and Problems
Bizarre Behavior, Violence, Substance Abuse, and Suicide

MANY OF THE SYMPTOMS and usual behaviors of people with schizophrenia or bipolar disorder are problematic. As you learn to understand them, they can become less disconcerting and more manageable. However, there are additional behaviors and symptoms that are even more worrisome to people close to those who are ill. While these behaviors may or may not be directly related to the illness, they may become dangerous to the ill person and others. In this chapter we discuss how to manage the potentially more serious situations in which the ill person engages in bizarre behavior, violence, substance abuse, and suicide attempts.

BIZARRE BEHAVIOR

People with mental illness may act in ways that are strange and unfamiliar to the rest of us. The first thing to consider when confronted with bizarre behavior is the degree of danger it presents. For example, some people with mental illness may have a ritual they perform before they sit in a chair or eat. They may be afraid to wear red or to be in a room with yellow walls or furniture. They may have unusual manner-isms or facial expressions. They may talk to themselves or laugh at inappropriate times. Such behaviors are harmless. They may be inconvenient or embarrassing to others, but it is extremely unlikely that these behaviors will ever hurt any-

DEALING WITH BIZARRE BEHAVIOR

Remember these basics about bizarre behavior:

- It is a symptom of an illness.
- You did not do anything to cause it.
- It is often related to delusional thinking.
- Ill people are sometimes able to control it.
- It usually does not present a danger to anyone.

Keep in mind the basic communication skills for deal-ing with a relative who has a mental illness. Especially:

1. Stay calm and nonjudgmental.
2. Be concise and direct in your statements.

Use the following guidelines in situations in which a relative is acting in a bizarre manner:

1. Decide what your limits are regarding your rela-tive's behavior both in private and in public places,

one. They are probably closely related to the symptoms of the illness—specifically, delusional thinking, poor judgment, or compulsive behavior.

Whenever possible, it is best to ignore such behaviors. Since they are harmless, and you usually have many other issues to deal with, it is not worthwhile spending time and energy on these behaviors. If the behaviors are particularly embarrassing or disturbing to you, you may want to ask your relative, in the

and communicate these when you and he or she are calm.

2. Decide, in advance, what the consequences will be if your relative exceeds the limits, and communicate these.

3. Follow through on the consequences when the situation calls for it.

4. If you are unfamiliar with the behavior, ask what the person is doing. If it relates to delusional thinking it is probably best not to pursue the content. Instead, calmly advise the person of the consequences of his or her behavior (if danger or police intervention is likely) or try to shift the focus to something constructive or more practical (if the behavior is relatively innocuous).

5. It is often wise to pay as little attention as possible to the bizarre behavior, focusing instead on positive, healthy activity and behavior.

manner described in chapter 3, to refrain from engaging in them while in your presence or in a public place. Some people are able to control these kinds of behaviors for limited periods of time. Keep in mind the possibility that your relative can do so only at those times when the symptoms are less severe.

The situation changes significantly when the behaviors

PREVENTING VIOLENCE

There are three general types of violent behavior, each requiring a different plan of response.

1. *A reaction to or expression of psychotic symptoms.* This type of violence is relatively rare. It is based purely on delusions and is not responsive to reasoning or discussion. People exhibiting such behavior should not be at home. Prompt police intervention or hospitalization is in order.

2. *Loss of self-control and subsequent lashing out.* When dealing with this type of violence:

   • Learn to recognize the cues related to your relative's losing control—for example, becoming wide-eyed or hyperventilating. This kind of violence is often evoked when a person feels cornered, threatened, or verbally attacked.

   • Stay calm, and convey your expectation that your relative will maintain control. Offer suggestions as to how he or she could best do this (going for a walk, putting the cup down, and so forth). Establish or reiterate limits.

pose a real danger to the ill person or to others. For example, a man may believe that in order to save the world from nuclear war, he has to run down the freeway naked; a woman may continue to borrow money from her gangster friend in a casino and have sexual encounters with all his friends to repay him; or a man may periodically get drunk, believe that

- Give as much emotional and physical distance as possible.
- Assure your own physical safety.
- After everyone has calmed down, discuss the incident. Underline its seriousness and the need for a plan to assure that it will not happen again.

3. *Gestures or threats of violence given primarily to control others or to get one's own way.* Handle these as follows:

- Evaluate the incident, both on your own and in conjunction with your relative.
- When everyone is calm, initiate a discussion outlining which behaviors are not acceptable and what their consequences will be. Your relative's wants and needs should also be considered.
- Be prepared to follow through on the consequences. These may include a loss of privileges or a call to police, depending on the seriousness of the behavior.

certain men are trying to turn him into a homosexual, and provoke physical fights with them.

In such situations, you may not be able to prevent the person from proceeding, but you do have several options. Your first is to advise your relative that you believe that what he or she intends to do is dangerous and will likely lead to his or her getting hurt and winding up in jail or a hospital. If this has happened in the past you would do well to remind the person of his or her previous experience. Avoid debating the merits or validity of what the person is doing or planning; focus on the consequences of the behavior in as calm a manner as possible.

If you feel that the situation is serious enough, you can set limits—saying, for example, that you will not continue to have contact with your relative or allow him or her to live with you if he or she chooses to engage in these dangerous activities. Sometimes practical considerations can override the demands of delusions, and people will be able to control their behavior in order to maintain their living situation or the much-needed contact and support of family and friends.

Your last resort, if your relative is in the process of doing something dangerous, is to call the police. Safety should outweigh the possible unpleasantness involved in dealing with the legal system. The Quick Reference Guide, Dealing with Bizarre Behavior on page 110, lists the key things to remember when you encounter bizarre behavior.

VIOLENCE

Violence is one of the most feared yet least likely behaviors of people with mental illness. While many people with mental illness act in unusual and unpredictable ways, they do not often strike out at someone. One of the best indicators of whether an individual has the potential to be violent is past history. If a person has never been violent, he or she is very unlikely to be so in the future.

However, if someone has been violent before, you need to examine the circumstances to determine if it might happen again. Was the person intoxicated? Psychotic? Completely out of control? Was the person taking medication? Did he or she feel threatened? Was the person provoked? Did he or she do harm to a person or property? The answers to these questions will help you determine the likelihood of future violence.

If, for example, your ill father was violent once, when he first became psychotic, but has since been taking medication for five years and has had no further incidents, it is unlikely that he will be violent again, especially while he is on medication. On the other hand, if your ill daughter recently be-

CYCLE OF VIOLENCE

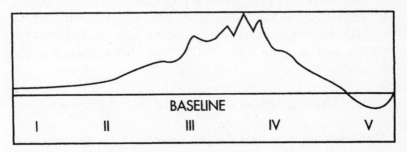

Phase I   Activation. Stress occurs, which may or may not be readily apparent.

Phase II   Escalation. Best time to intervene.

Phase III   Crisis. Violence occurs.

Phase IV   Recovery. Still agitated, but less emotional and less physical.

Phase V   Stabilization. Guilt, remorse; person ready to discuss and listen to interventions.

came violent rather suddenly while on medication because a voice told her to punch someone, it is possible that she could strike out again.

The Quick Reference Guide entitled Preventing Violence on page 112 outlines three types of violent behavior and how to handle them.

The preceding chart shows that for most incidents of violence there is a distinguishable beginning, middle, and end. Keeping this in mind may provide some comfort immediately following the violence. The chart also allows you to consider where you are in the cycle and when it is best to intervene.

In all cases your safety must be protected. If you believe you are in danger and the ill person is unable to control himself or herself, you must remove yourself from the situation and/or call the police. Even if the violence is directed exclusively at property, it should be dealt with seriously, with significant consequences enforced, including repairing or paying for the damages. Some people are able to limit themselves to violence against property; others commit more indiscriminately violent acts. It is not wise to allow any form of violence.

SUBSTANCE ABUSE OR CHEMICAL DEPENDENCY

Those people who have both a mental illness and a serious problem with drugs or alcohol have far more than twice the difficulties of people who have either one alone. The best-known treatment approach for each problem acts in opposition to the best-known approach for the other. There are extremely few outstanding treatment programs that deal effectively with both a major mental illness and a serious substance-abuse problem.

Programs for people with mental illness tend to provide warm, supportive environments. They foster as much independence as possible, while providing ways to meet clients' basic needs when they are unable to do so for themselves. Chemical-dependency recovery programs tend to be extremely confrontational. They are highly structured and utilize discipline systems that are sometimes based on shame and humiliation. The coping mechanisms of many people who abuse substances include manipulating, lying, stealing, and other antisocial behaviors. These people tend to take advantage of people who have schizophrenia or severe affective disorders. Neither group tends to feel very comfortable with the other.

In the past, someone who had both problems would often bounce back and forth between programs designed to serve one problem or the other. Programs for drug and alcohol abuse typically do not allow their clients to take any form of medication. They may help a person with mental illness temporarily get a handle on alcoholism, but since that person cannot take psychiatric medication, the symptoms of his or her mental illness soon flair up. He or she winds up back in a psychiatric hospital. There the person might be stabilized on medication again, only to begin drinking and thus starting the cycle all over.

Since the mid 1980s there has been an explosion in the number of people with both a serious mental illness and a substance-abuse problem. Although no one is entirely sure why this has occurred, one reason may be that since there are fewer people with mental illness in institutions, more of these people have access to drugs and alcohol. Another reason may be that people with mental illness have a greater need to medicate and numb themselves with drugs and alcohol now that they are faced with the prejudice and stigma outside institutions and with the shortage of housing and treatment programs. Whatever the cause, mental-health workers now face the challenge of figuring out what to do about the situation.

Mental-health professionals and drug and alcohol counselors have traditionally been at odds with one another. Only in more recent years have they begun to join forces and recognize that, in dealing with people with a dual diagnosis, there are benefits to be derived from many different kinds of programs. How to best design treatment programs to address both problems in depth has yet to be determined.

Unfortunately, this situation means that families and friends are often left to handle the problems themselves—a double burden, and more than double the work. They must

DEALING WITH SUBSTANCE ABUSE

What constitutes alcoholism or substance abuse? Although there are various definitions, most professionals agree that substance abuse exists when a person's functioning is adversely affected as a result of drinking or using drugs. Any one of the following may occur:

1. deterioration of family relationships—for example, divorce, suspended contact with family
2. multiple arrests (including arrests for drunk driving)
3. evidence of related physical/medical problems
4. loss of job or living situation, or expulsion from a treatment program

Families can help in the following ways:

1. Talk about the problem and your concern. Denial is almost always a major barrier that alcoholics and drug abusers have to overcome before recovery or treatment is possible. Do not go along with the denial. Give concrete examples of the

educate themselves about dealing not only with mental illness but also with substance abuse.

When people have a problem with drugs or alcohol, it needs to be confronted directly. The first line of defense for addicts and alcoholics is to deny, minimize, or attempt to rationalize away the problem. They will explain how they don't have a problem at all, that if they do have a problem it is well under control, or that the problem is so minimal it is not

negative effects of abuse that you have seen in your relative's life.

2. Recognize the magnitude of the undertaking involved in trying to give up a chemical dependence or addiction. It is a long, slow process. Eventually people have to develop a new way of life and new ways to cope with all the difficult feelings they were using the drugs or alcohol to escape from.

3. Encourage your relative to accept the problem. This is the first major step. Support all of his or her efforts to seek help or to stop using the substance.

4. Encourage your relative to attend support groups like Alcoholics Anonymous. These groups provide a very effective method for recovery.

5. Understand that most people have slips or relapses during recovery, and make sure your relative understands this, too.

6. Participate in Al-Anon, CoDA (Co-dependents Anonymous), or other support groups for families of alcoholics or addicts.

worth bothering about. It is up to you to disagree and to point out why you feel they have a problem and need help.

In spite of what most addicts and alcoholics believe, very few can successfully deal with a serious drug or alcohol problem by themselves. They usually need to obtain help as well as make major changes in their lives. Theirs is a long, slow journey, best undertaken with a lot of support from people who are going through a similar process. Family members need lots of support as well. They need to look at what part they may have played in the addiction process and how to change certain aspects of their behavior.

The problem is further complicated by the fact that drugs and alcohol, and the symptoms of mental illness significantly impact one another. People who have a major mental illness are at far greater risk of abusing drugs and alcohol than those without a mental illness. Compared with people who have either a mental illness or a substance-use disorder, people with both often experience more severe and chronic medical, social, and emotional problems. They are also more likely to be violent than those with a mental illness alone. Because they have two disorders, they are more vulnerable to both psychiatric and substance-abuse relapses. Relapse in substance use often leads to psychiatric symptom relapse. Similarly, increase in psychiatric symptoms often leads to relapse in substance use. Thus, it is especially important for those with a dual diagnosis to learn, and for their families to understand, relapse-prevention skills. It is also vital for consumers and families to understand the interaction of medication with alcohol and drugs of abuse.

Few people will readily admit to having either a mental illness or a drug or alcohol problem. Acknowledging both serious problems can take a long time, both for the people afflicted and their families. If you suspect that your relative with a mental illness has a substance-abuse problem as well, pay close attention to the Quick Reference Guide entitled Dealing with Substance Abuse on page 118, and the last chapter. Substance abuse is a serious and potentially life-threatening problem that won't disappear if you ignore it. You must face it directly and learn how to deal with it.

SUICIDE

Suicide is one of the most feared yet least talked about aspects of mental illness. Many families live in constant dread that their loved one may resort to suicide. Unfortunately, most families are not able to discuss suicide openly and so do not learn to recognize its indicators and possible interventions they can make.

The sad truth is that the rate of suicide is about twelve times higher among people with mental illness than among the population at large. About 10 percent of people with major mental illnesses do ultimately kill themselves. It is not surprising that the rate is so high when you consider how difficult the lives of people with mental illness are.

There are several reasons that people with mental illness kill themselves. The most common cause of suicide has as much to do with the secondary symptoms of the illness as it does with the illness itself. Many people make a conscious decision to end their lives because they are extremely unhappy with their situation. These people are able to think clearly enough to know that they are ill and that they may be so for many years. They realize how limited and painful their lives are and cannot bear the thought of continuing with them.

While we may be tempted to judge these people harshly, it is impossible for us to know how we might react if faced with the sometimes torturous symptoms of a mental illness and the isolation, alienation, and rejection with which this country reacts to people who have a mental illness. Setting

PREVENTING SUICIDE

Someone's likelihood of suicide is usually expressed in terms of the following categories (listed in order of increasing seriousness).

1. *Ideation*: thoughts or feelings about killing oneself, without any immediate plan or intention of acting on them.

2. *Gestures*: self-destructive acts that a person connects with suicidal thoughts or feelings (taking ten aspirins, dropping a typewriter on one's foot). These are often seen as an effort to communicate (for example, a cry for help), to which a response should be made.

3. *Attempts*: a wide range of actions in terms of lethality.

Warning signs of suicide include the following:

1. Movement into or out of a depression if the person:

   - exhibits feelings of extreme worthlessness or expresses concerns about having committed an unpardonable sin.

   - expresses utter hopelessness about the future and shows a lack of desire to make any future plans.

   - hears voices instructing him or her to hurt or kill himself or herself.

   - exhibits a sudden change in mood from severe depression to inexplicable brightness or serenity.

- gets his or her affairs in order—for example, writes a will or systematically contacts old friends and relatives.

- discusses a concrete, specific suicidal plan.

2. Talking about having supernatural powers, being indestructible, and so forth while in a manic or delusional state.

3. Previous suicidal gestures or attempts or extreme impulsivity, combined with any of the above.

Preventative measures and appropriate responses include the following:

1. Any suicidal talk or actions should be taken seriously; they warrant attention, even if there may be little likelihood that the person will hurt or kill himself or herself.

2. If the person is severely depressed, do not ignore, minimize, or deny his or her feelings, but rather empathize ("It must be terrible to feel that way") and offer emotional support and encouragement for any recent accomplishments. You may assure your relative that feelings of depression and despair are common among people who have serious emotional or mental problems and that they will most likely lessen over time.

3. If the person appears to be preparing for suicide, try to determine if he or she has a specific plan. The closer the person is to having one, the more you might want to:

continued on following page

continued from previous page

- Seek professional help and/or encourage him or her to do the same.
- Try to elicit an agreement that the person will not act on these feelings without first contacting you, a mental-health crisis hotline in your area such as Suicide Prevention, his or her doctor, or another responsible person.
- Secure any possible weapons (razors, knives, pills) the person might have available and be inclined to use.

4. If your relative is delusional, get immediate help.

5. It is important to distinguish for yourself and your relative the difference between thoughts, feelings, and actions. Thinking or feeling like killing oneself is very different from actually doing something self-destructive. When in doubt, call a suicide prevention service, the police, or the local psychiatric emergency services for a phone consultation.

6. Some suicides happen with no warning. Nothing anyone can do will prevent them.

aside any judgments about whether people have the right to take their own lives, it is certainly understandable that people who have suffered so much might want to put an end to their pain. They sometimes feel there is no other way to do this.

Other people, more seriously ill than the ones discussed above, kill themselves as a direct result of their symptoms. They are psychotic at the time, and do not believe that they will die. For example, a person in the midst of a manic episode may believe that he or she has superhuman powers or is indestructible. The person may consequently decide to race a car off a cliff or dive into freezing cold water. Another may believe he or she is on a mission from God when jumping in front of a train. Such people may not realize the consequences of their behavior, or may feel compelled to do things that their voices dictate. They may feel a need to exorcise the evil they think is within them and not realize that the exorcism could kill them. These are perhaps the saddest kinds of suicides, because these people probably do not want to end their lives.

Lastly, some people kill themselves unintentionally, while trying to communicate something else. They may have wanted attention, hospitalization, or temporary relief from the symptoms, but by taking too many pills, driving too fast, or cutting their wrists they end their lives by accident. Rather than being delusional, they may be overcome with intolerable emotions and unable to ask directly for help.

If your relative displays any indication of thinking about suicide, or makes a suicide gesture or attempt, do not hesitate to talk about it, being careful to do so compassionately. If you feel unable to do so, then help him or her connect with someone who can. Families are often reluctant to broach the topic for fear of increasing the likelihood that their relative will make a suicide attempt. The opposite is more likely to be true. Not talking about suicidal feelings, the reasons behind them, and possible alternatives, may leave the person feeling they have no other choice. There is nothing wrong with asking your son if he is thinking of taking his life or hurting himself when there is evidence to suggest he may be having such thoughts. However, you want to be careful not to ask frequently if he repeatedly says he has no such thoughts or feelings.

The Quick Reference Guide on page 122, Preventing Suicide, summarizes how to assess the likelihood of someone's committing suicide; it also lists some early warning signs and suggests preventative measures that you can take.

Families and friends are profoundly affected by the suicide of a loved one with a mental illness. A mixture of feelings often follows. People may feel sad and guilty, wishing they had done something to prevent the death. It is amazing how many people feel responsible for a suicide after it occurs. Every friend, relative, and professional involved with the ill person may think he or she could have prevented the death by doing one or two things differently. More often than not, however, no one could have prevented it. The choice and responsibility ultimately rest with the people who kill themselves. If a person is determined to die, there is nothing anyone can do to stop him or her. People have committed suicide in the most secure locked facilities our society knows how to build.

Many people also struggle with anger after suicide. They may feel angry with mental-health professionals for not preventing the death or offering more or better services. They may feel angry with the person for killing himself or herself and inflicting such pain on loved ones. It is not surprising that anger follows such an irreversible act—one that friends and family had no control over and wish had not been chosen.

At the same time family and friends frequently feel some sense of relief as well. Neither the person who was ill nor family and friends have to suffer anymore. It is quite normal and understandable to feel relief that you and your loved one are no longer in pain. It is often the end of a long and excruciating struggle for everyone involved. It is a tragic end to a tragic life.

If your relative does commit suicide or make a serious attempt, you must find ways to deal with all your feelings. You must talk about them or get special support for yourself. There are books and counselors available for people grieving a loss by suicide. You will only increase your pain and suffering if you choose to deal with the trauma alone.

6

Coping with
Your Own Feelings

SEEING SOMEONE YOU LOVE suffer from a major mental illness is an extremely painful, frightening, confusing, and infuriating experience. Since the nature of the illness is such that the symptoms may come and go unpredictably, you never know what to expect. You will likely experience a wide range of emotions—from hope to anger to extreme sadness to wondering "Why me?" to wishing that your life could have been as normal as that of so many people you know.

This chapter explores the many common concerns and feelings of parents, siblings, children, and friends of people with mental illness and offers suggestions as to how to deal with problems that some of these feelings bring. Just as it is crucial to have an understanding of what the world of mental illness is like, it is important to understand and acknowledge what *your* world is like. Rest assured that you are not alone in feeling and thinking all that you do about your relative and your life.

It is not fair that so many good, loving people have their lives devastated by severe illnesses. This injustice can shake even the most firmly held belief about religion, morality, and the meaning of life. It is indeed an incredible challenge to try to integrate the pain and suffering you see and feel with a more hopeful worldview. People can spend years trying to understand why such a terrible thing happened to their family, attempting to find some meaning or make some sense out of a situation that makes no sense at all. It is just a matter of luck that some families have to deal with this horror and others do not. If often takes years to resolve or accept such inequities in life.

Unfortunately, many families feel embarrassed or ashamed about mental illness, as if it were some reflection on them. This is especially true of children who have an ill parent and teenagers who have an ill sibling. At a young age we are particularly sensitive to what other people think of us and those close to us. Children want to believe that their parents and siblings are wonderful. When a close relative acts in obviously bizarre ways it can be devastating to a child. The situation can also thrust children into the position of needing to assume adult responsibilities long before they are ready. This can lead to problems when they become adults.

Underlying this issue is the difficulty our culture has in accepting people who are different. Most of us do not do well with people who have different ideas, who look different, or who have a mental illness and may therefore act different. We may be frightened by them or treat them as outcasts or second-class citizens. It is unfortunate that we have not been taught to hold mental illness in the same regard as we hold heart disease, diabetes, or other illnesses. People rarely feel ashamed of having a relative with heart disease.

Relatives of people with mental illness often grow to dread the ringing of the telephone. They never know who may be calling. Perhaps it is the ill relative asking for more money or venting anger for no apparent reason, or perhaps it is the police, the hospital, or a crisis unit. The list of possibilities seems endless. None of them brings good news.

Over time many people who have been dealing with a loved one with a mental illness may even get to the point of feeling they cannot go on. They feel like they are walking on eggshells, never knowing what might set the ill person off. Some families who have tried everything, to no avail, become exhausted and feel they must change their phone number, move away, or end all contact. They may become so exasperated that they wish the ill person would simply disappear or even die.

While no one feels good about wishing for the death of a loved one, this is a common and eminently understandable reaction. To watch someone you love gradually or episodically slip away is a torturous process; it makes sense to wish for its end. This does not mean that you don't love your relative, but that you are experiencing enormous pain and feel helpless to put an end to your suffering and that of your relative. It more closely resembles the wish for a mercy killing than any indication of a lack of caring. More important, beneath it also lies the lost hope for an end to the pain and for the ill person's complete recovery.

Unfortunately, people often turn some of these feelings against themselves and those closest to them. The pain eats away at those family members who secretly feel guilty and blame themselves for what has happened to their relative. If we could get a nickel for every sleepless night spent by a relative of a person with a mental illness, we would probably have enough money to find a cure. Many people talk of waking in the middle of the night blaming themselves for not having done things differently, thinking they could have prevented the illness. They spend hours on *what ifs*: "What if I had insisted on getting him out of the class of that second-grade teacher he hated? Maybe then he wouldn't have become ill."

Or worse, "If only her father had been gentler on her, then . . ." Later in this chapter I will discuss guilt and offer some suggestions on how to handle these feelings.

Families resent the disruption that mental illness brings to their lives. Parents who were looking forward to retiring with fewer responsibilities have a forty-year-old ill child still dependent on them; an adult daughter has to take care of her ill mother in addition to her own children; a young girl has an ill brother who continues to demand most of her parents' time, energy, and financial reserves. All these people are continuously reminded of the impact mental illness has on their lives.

Social misconceptions also spill over to your interactions with friends and relatives, who are far too eager to give you advice, much of it misguided, about how to handle your relative. They imply or state explicitly that you caused the problems or perpetuate them. The uncle who tells you that you ought to be more strict or the teacher who tells you that you were too strict, the preacher who tells you to do more for your relative or the grandparent who tells you that you do too much—though each may have good intentions, none has any idea how much he or she adds to your pain, doubts, and fears about what part you may have played in your relative's illness.

Living with someone who has a mental illness, or having such a person in your life, inevitably gives rise to a vast array of feelings. Some of these may lessen as you learn how to handle stress and how to deal more effectively with your ill relative. However, it is of the utmost importance to keep in mind that none of your feelings is inappropriate. By acknowledging this you can avoid the unnecessary pain brought on by feelings of guilt for your own anger, frustration, and discouragement. What follows is a description of some of the more difficult reactions healthy families and friends have, and suggestions for how to cope with them. It is okay to make mistakes; only by making mistakes will you know what works with your ill relative. If you are not making mistakes, you are probably not exploring all the possibilities.

THE GRIEVING PROCESS

When someone first displays the symptoms of a mental illness, those around that person usually become confused and upset. Suddenly or gradually, they see their loved one behaving and talking in strange and different ways that make no sense. They may think that the unusual behavior is a phase, part of adolescence, a reaction to drugs, or a response to stress. But as the symptoms persist, they see the personality of someone they love completely transformed, and their fear, anxiety, concern, and pain increase.

The initial reaction of most of us to a loved one's diagnosis of any severe, chronic, or life-threatening illness is shock and denial. We think it impossible that someone who was recently healthy and happy has suddenly received a long-term sentence of pain. We may not believe for days, weeks, months, or even years that this has happened. Everything may feel unreal for a while. We may walk around dazed, thinking, "This can't be happening to me, to my family."

Most people also feel enormous sadness. Those who can cry do so a lot. Those who cannot cry carry their pain inside. We feel the tragedy of having the life of a loved one devastated. It is especially painful for parents to watch their child, a promising young adult, be struck down in his or her prime. They see their child's life becoming so much less than they wanted. They have lost, for all practical purposes, the son or daughter they once had. Yet they are reminded of their child's previous potential at times just by seeing him, especially when he feels a little better and seems more like he used to be. Siblings too often feel a particular kind of loss when the older sister or brother they used to love and perhaps look up to is no longer able to function well and has changed in many other ways.

Lastly, there is usually a great deal of frustration and anger that comes with the helplessness we feel in our inability to lessen the symptoms of the illness. Sometimes this anger gets directed at the mental-health system, and at the government agencies that do not allocate enough money for treatment and research for mental illness. This is one of the most productive places to direct anger, especially if the result is an effort to change our government's priorities. Unfortunately, the anger is more often directed at the ill person or those family members who may have differing ideas about how to handle the situation. Many family arguments focus on how to handle the ill person or the latest crisis.

The feelings described above—denial, sadness, and anger—are actually part of the natural grieving process and are typical reactions people have to any major loss. Major mental illness does constitute an enormous loss. The person as you knew her or him before may seldom be around again. You must allow yourself to grieve this loss.

Most people in this country have a difficult time grieving, or being with others who are grieving a loss by death. When someone dies or when an important relationship ends, we usually go in and out of denial, depression, and anger until we eventually come to accept the loss. This process is much more difficult for relatives of people with mental illness, because there is not the same finality. The person seems gone; then, when the symptoms abate, the person seems to be back, at least partially. You inevitably get your hopes up, only to have them dashed again when the symptoms worsen once more. It is like being on an endless emotional roller coaster. Just when you have accepted things the way they are, they change. The unpredictability and ever-changing severity of the symptoms cause families a great deal of pain.

Grieving is, however, a necessary part of the process of learning to live with a relative who has a serious mental illness. It takes time to go through the denial, anger, sadness, and depression that accompany losing someone near and dear. Indeed, it usually takes longer than you would like, longer than you think it will, and longer than you think it should.

COPING WITH STRESS

The feelings and situations that families of people with mental illness experience add up to a great deal of additional stress. Indeed, families and friends of people with mental illness often find themselves with headaches and stomach problems. They may have difficulty sleeping, eating, or socializing, and may experience all the other common physical manifestations of stress.

The stress of mental illness can and does tear many families apart. There are, unfortunately, many divorces among parents of people with mental illness. People often have very strong and differing opinions about the best way to handle things, how involved to be, and how much to take care of the person versus how much to encourage the person to take care of himself or herself.

Researchers have devised a scale for measuring stress. Different events were assigned ratings according to the amount of stress they usually cause. Not surprisingly, many of the events high on the stress scale occur in families having a relative who has a mental illness. Following are some of the categories that often apply to friends and relatives of people with a mental illness:

- change in health or behavior
- change in financial state
- change in number of arguments with spouse
- sexual difficulties
- son or daughter leaving home
- in-law troubles
- change in living conditions
- change in personal habits
- change in recreational habits
- change in sleeping habits
- change in eating habits

WORKSHEET FOR HANDLING YOUR OWN STRESS

Identify three situations that create stress in your life.

1. _____

2. _____

3. _____

During each of these situations, how do you feel (anxious, depressed, irritable, angry, headachy, and so forth)?

1. _____

2. _____

3. _____

- change in family get-togethers
- marital separation

Learning to successfully cope with stress involves several important steps. You must learn first what causes you to feel stress; second, how you react under stress; and finally, what helps you feel better. Without finding ways to cope with stress, you and other family members will be unable to offer the kind of quality support your ill relative needs.

It would be like giving an exhausted and distraught carpenter his or her tools and asking him or her to build some cabinets. You would no sooner want to live with those cabi-

---

Now think of what feels comforting or nurturing to you during these times (exercising, hibernating, talking to a friend, going away, meditating, watching TV).

1. _____
2. _____
3. _____

You need to build comforting things into your routine. It is important to know and respect your own limits regarding how much stress you can tolerate, including the stress of dealing with your ill relative. It is normal to want to take breaks or vacations from dealing with your relative. The chances are high that when you return you will be better able to deal with your relative, and with your own stress as well.

nets than you would with the results of your interaction with someone with a mental illness when you are depleted and angry. The Quick Reference Guide entitled Worksheet for Handling Your Own Stress can help you find ways to cope with your stress.

People with mental illness need their family's love and support. These can significantly improve the quality of their lives and reduce the amount of suffering they experience. However, the only way a family can offer love and support is by devoting time and energy to keeping the rest of the family as strong, healthy, and happy as possible. In the long run, a little bit of quality time with an ill relative goes much further than daily visits that are resented and leave you drained and depleted.

It is not easy to focus on yourself and healthy family members when your ill relative has so much less than the others. After all, he or she may be unable to take vacations or has little joy in life. You must keep reminding yourself that your relative's life does not improve when you deprive yourself. The person will benefit from your being in his or her life only if you are available in a nurturing, loving, supportive manner. You can offer this only if you provide yourself with nurturing and support.

Taking care of yourself means doing fun things without the ill person. You must take vacations on your own, and have separate interests, activities, and friends. You must learn to allow yourself some distance from the ill relative. If you cannot do that, you will never be able to offer the kind of love and support he or she needs. While your relative needs to learn to live as full a life as he or she can, he or she also needs *you* to live as full a life as you can.

Although people who have a mental illness may often seem unaware of what is going on around them, they are usually acutely aware of the emotional climate. They are probably very tuned in to how you are feeling and how your life is going. Many people who have a mental illness feel very guilty about how their illness has changed the lives of their families. Though most cannot clearly articulate these feelings, they feel relieved when others continue to lead their own lives. The Quick Reference Guide entitled Keeping a Life of Your Own can serve as a reminder of the importance of fortifying yourself through the ordeal of having a relative with a mental illness.

You must learn how to pace yourself. Living your life is like running a constant marathon. Unless you continue to replenish yourself and go at a speed your body can tolerate, you will collapse. Many families put all else on the back burner in order to do everything possible for their ill relative. When nothing produces the results they want, they turn their backs on their ill relative.

Just as people's tolerance for running a marathon will vary, the amount of time, energy, money, and contact people can offer a relative with a mental illness varies. Respect your own limits; you may wish you were the kind of person who could see your ill relative every week and comfortably have him or her to your house for the holidays. But if you are able to offer only a phone call twice a month, this is better in the long run, for both of you, than trying to do more than you can. The quality of the contact will be worth a great deal more than any greater quantity that comes with resentment.

It is equally important to respect the pace of others in your family. Their pace may be different from yours; it may be different from what you would like it to be. This often leads to arguments and tension. You have enough to handle with your ill relative. If you can accept the differences in people's tolerance for dealing with mental illness, you will avoid unnecessary additional stress in your life. It is easy to think that others are wrong or bad because they do not do things the way you would like them to. Yet only by accepting differing opinions and paces will you be able to have the harmony and support you need within your family.

The Value of Educating Yourself

Family members usually do their best to deal with mental illness; with education and support their best can be greatly improved. Education is one of the most crucial survival tools for dealing with these confusing and complicated illnesses. The symptoms are difficult to recognize, especially in the beginning. The treatments can also be confusing. The mental-health system itself, and all the legal procedures involved, are extremely complex and, at times, illogical. Without a good

KEEPING A LIFE OF YOUR OWN

Sometimes it seems impossible, in the midst of the day-by-day trauma of dealing with a relative with a serious mental illness, to keep your own hopes, ambitions, and sense of accomplishment alive. However, the more difficult such an undertaking may seem, the more important it is to strive to do just that. Here are ten ways you can deal with the despair and depression brought on by your relative's illness, limitations, and pain.

1. Participate in activities that are yours alone—for example, working, going to the theater, talking with friends, going on vacation.

2. Remember that having your own life will increase your relative's respect for you.

working knowledge of these, your life will be much more frustrating and overwhelming. Even if you do understand them all, you will have reason to be angry, frustrated, pained, and bewildered.

Mental illnesses are often unpredictable. You must learn to expect the unexpected. You can save yourself enormous wear and tear if you learn from a friendly instructor or counselor rather than from ten years in the school of hard knocks. By reading, by watching or listening to tapes, or by taking classes you can start to recognize the signs that indicate that your relative is starting to become more ill. Early intervention can save everyone unnecessary pain and suffering. Similarly, education can help you notice when your relative is making

3. Remember that your inner resources are greater than you generally imagine.

4. Accept the limits of what you can do for and give to your relative.

5. Accept the reality of your relative's illness and limitations without blaming yourself or others.

6. Learn to expect the unpredictable and unexpected.

7. Continue to educate yourself and others and get support.

8. Strive for good physical health by means of a good diet and sufficient exercise. Do things to reduce your stress level.

9. Make efforts to maintain social contacts.

10. Give support, time, and energy to others in situations similar to your own.

some significant progress. Because progress often occurs at a much slower pace than we would like, it can easily be over-looked.

Become familiar with the mental-health services available in your area. Whether or not your relative is currently inter-ested in using them, it is important for you to know about them. The most difficult time to do anything is in the middle of a crisis. The sooner you learn where to turn when there is a crisis or when your relative decides he or she wants some help, the better equipped you will be to handle such situations. The wisest, most prepared families have the phone numbers and addresses of psychiatric emergency services, doctors, and so forth conveniently located near their phone. Anything you can do to end a crisis a few minutes sooner will be a godsend in the heat of the moment.

NAMI (formerly The National Alliance for the Mentally Ill)

The best source in the United States for the ongoing edu-cation and support you will need is the National Alliance for the Mentally Ill. This group was organized in 1979 by fami-lies frustrated with the lack of services, treatment, research, and education available for people with mental illness and their families. It has become the nation's largest and most im-portant source of advocacy for people with mental illness. It is now a growing alliance of families, mental-health profes-sionals, and consumers of mental-health services. Chapters vary in how frequently they meet and in exactly which serv-ices they provide. But you can count on finding friendly, un-derstanding people who have had experiences very similar to your own. Often they can provide, or tell you where to find, the help you will need for yourself and for your relative. Many groups offer family support groups and educational programs. Some have hotlines for you to call in crises or moments of uncertainty and pain. Some offer referrals to competent doctors, as well as to relevant housing, food, and treatment programs. NAMI is the best vehicle for working to increase the appropriations of government funds for mental illness and to change related legislation. The national headquarters are located in Arlington, Virginia. There are local chapters, called "affiliates," in almost every city and county in the country. NAMI has more than 220,000 members, with 1,200 state and local affiliates in all fifty states, the District of Columbia, Puerto Rico, American Samoa, and Canada. You are strongly encouraged to contact a local, state, or national office, join the organization, and begin receiving their very informative newsletters. You can obtain contact information in your local telephone directory, through the national office phone number 1-800-950-6264, or on their website: *www.NAMI.org.*

Having a supportive place to talk and learn about mental illness can be the most important thing for your own sanity. With few people understanding what you are going through, and fewer still knowing *how* to be there for you, there is nothing quite like talking with others who have been through it before you. Joining a support group may be one of the most comforting things you can do for yourself.

There is a great deal to learn about mental illness and how to handle someone with a mental illness. It will take time to learn how to deal with all the feelings you and other family members will have. You need to learn to be as patient with yourself as you are with your ill relative. Just as you must learn what you can realistically expect from your ill relative, you must also learn what you can realistically expect from yourself. The Quick Reference Guide, Realistic Goals and Expectations for Yourself, summarizes goals you want to strive toward. Be aware that it will take some people longer than others to achieve them.

REALISTIC GOALS AND EXPECTATIONS
FOR YOURSELF

Educate yourself. Learn about the illness and how to cope with it to the best of your abilities.

Develop your ability to respond to your relative in a calm and considered, rather than reactive, way.

Become increasingly able to recognize and appreciate small signs of improvement.

Become increasingly able to recognize signs of deterioration without a great deal of panic.

Become increasingly able to enjoy and enrich the quality of your own life, in spite of the tragedy in your family.

Improve your ability to keep a loving distance from your relative's life.

Continue to seek the support you need in order to do all of the above.

SPECIAL CONCERNS OF SIBLINGS AND CHILDREN

While mental illness seriously affects everyone in a family, each member's reactions will differ somewhat. Often siblings or children of a person with a mental illness may try to distance themselves from the situation as soon as they can and may act as if it is not their concern. Nonetheless, the family member's illness is usually a traumatic part of their childhood, and the consequent scars and worries may permeate their lives for years. In their young adulthood they often fear becoming ill themselves. As they grow older and have families of their own they worry about their children becoming ill. It is important that they familiarize themselves with the statistics presented in chapter 1 so they will know just how likely this is. Some may want to talk with a genetic counselor to ascertain how the statistics apply to them. Many siblings back away from the entire issue (much to their parents' dismay) and let their parents handle all the problems with their ill brother or sister. However, these siblings live in anxious anticipation of the day their parents are no longer alive. They know that they may then feel compelled to handle the problems.

Having a parent or sibling who has a mental illness can interfere with the normal developmental process. Special support or therapy may be necessary later in life to assist in the processing of the experience if the necessary education and understanding are not available while the family is in the midst of the experience.

People's limits and tolerance for being with someone who is ill or disabled vary greatly. For many it takes days to recover from the pain of seeing someone suffer. It is best if everyone can respect these differences. It takes different amounts of time and a degree of maturity before someone is ready to involve himself or herself with an ill relative. The Quick Reference Guide, Growing Up with a Relative Who Has a Mental Illness, summarizes the particular issues with which siblings and children of people with mental illness struggle.

GUILT

Almost all relatives of people with mental illness feel guilty about their relative's life or their own. These feelings range from low-grade nagging background guilt to a pervasive, devastating condition. Guilt about an ill relative has no ra-

GROWING UP WITH A RELATIVE
WHO HAS A MENTAL ILLNESS

Siblings and children of people with a mental illness most commonly experience:

- denial
- confusion
- shame
- sadness
- guilt
- fear
- frustration
- anger
- resentment

Having a parent or sibling with a mental illness often interferes with or significantly impacts:

- social relationships
- one's image of one's family
- relationships with one's parents
- one's choice of activities and responsibilities
- one's emotional well-being

The most difficult times occur:

1. at the onset of the illness

2. during adolescence
3. during episodes when the ill relative is acutely ill and behaves in ways that are especially strange, unpredictable, and unacceptable

Things that help include:

1. a family that is open to discussing the illness and its effects on everyone
2. supportive relationships with people with whom one can talk about the situation
3. learning about the illness, especially about how likely it is that one or one's children will become ill
4. focusing on one's own activities and relationships

How much and what kind of impact an illness will have on a sibling is affected by whether the ill person:

- is older or younger
- is of the same or the opposite sex
- is close in age
- has a very severe or unpredictable illness

Many siblings and adult children of people with a mental illness cope with the problems by distancing themselves from the family and from the ill person for varying periods of time.

tional basis. It seems a part of human nature to feel responsible for those we love and for everything that happens to them. There is a part of each of us that never entirely outgrows the infantile sense that we are the center of the universe and have magically caused all that happens in our lives—

GUILT

Nearly all relatives of people with mental illness feel guilty, at some point, about their relative's or their own situation. Although it may never completely disappear, the feeling can be significantly reduced.

Causes of guilt:

1. blaming yourself or regretting your feelings (especially anger), thoughts, or actions regarding your ill relative
2. feeling bad about having a better life than your relative does (survivor guilt)
3. society's ostracism of families who have a relative with a mental illness

Effects of guilt:

1. depression; lack of energy for the present
2. dwelling on the past
3. diminished self-confidence and self-worth
4. less effectiveness in solving problems and achieving goals

especially the bad things. These feelings may lie dormant until a tragedy occurs. Then they come out in full force.

Another kind of guilt that affects relatives of people with any severe or disabling illness is called *survivor guilt*. This is the feeling that we do not deserve to have a better life than

> 5. acting like a martyr, in an effort to make up for past sins
> 6. being overprotective, which leads to your relative's feeling more helpless and dependent
> 7. diminished quality of your life
>
> *Deal with guilt by developing more rational and less painful ways of thinking about the situation.*
>
> 1. Acknowledge and express your guilt with an understanding listener.
> 2. Examine the beliefs underlying your guilt. (For example: "I should have done things differently when he was a child"; "I should have noticed the signs sooner and done something to prevent it"; "I should never have said that to her."
> 3. Counteract these false beliefs, using the information you have learned about the causes and course of mental illness.
> 4. Try not to dwell on the past.
> 5. Focus on how you may improve the present and the future for yourself and your ill relative.
> 6. Remind yourself that you deserve a good life even if your relative may not be fortunate enough to have one.

those near and dear to us. It is the flip side of wondering why terrible things happen to good people. We may struggle with the issue of why we can have complete lives when others cannot. There is no simple answer to any of these questions, but a practical approach to dealing with them is outlined in The Quick Reference Guide entitled Guilt.

Because guilt can significantly interfere with your ability to live a full life, talking with an understanding listener can be vital if your feelings are strong and disruptive. Keeping such feelings bottled up will only make them and their effects worse. Once you identify the false beliefs behind guilt, you can begin to argue more rationally with them. This, of course, presumes that you have educated yourself about mental illnesses—another important reason to seek such education.

Developing new ways of thinking about the situation takes time, patience, and a willingness to learn and to discuss your situation with others. This may be difficult, for two reasons. Some people believe that problems need to be handled solely within the family whenever possible. They think it weak or wrong to ask for outside help. This approach leads to a great deal of unnecessary suffering for many families. No one person or family needs to deal with any tragedy alone. It is impossible for families to handle complicated illnesses effectively without education and support.

Secondly, our culture's prejudice and ignorance about mental illness also make it difficult for many families to seek help. It is important for them to find people who are sympathetic to families struggling with mental illness. Such people will treat the situation much as they would that of someone who suddenly becomes blind or gets cancer. They rally whatever support and comfort they can. Unfortunately, most people are not so understanding, and tend to shy away or to feed the family's fears and feelings of guilt.

The saddest thing about guilt is its tenaciousness. Even families who have read all the books about mental illness and know all there is to know about the biological causes do not always rest easy. They, too, report that they wake in the middle of the night plagued by irrational questions about how they might have done things differently.

While it may not be possible for all families to completely rid themselves of nagging doubts, it is important to keep such doubts in perspective. Remind yourself that letting them prevail will certainly detract from what you can do to improve your relative's life today. Those who dwell on the past become too distracted to provide much help in the present, and this, ironically, provides more to feel guilty about in the future. What works best is for each family member to live as fully as possible in the present, to give as much as he or she can, and to avoid dwelling on the unanswerable. This is a long-term goal, much easier to formulate than to achieve.

ANGER AND FRUSTRATION

Anger and frustration also frequently plague families and friends of people with mental illness. This is especially true when families and friends first encounter the symptoms, before they understand what is going on. Anger and frustration may also persist when these people recognize the limitations of the mental-health system and their own inability to effect any significant changes. No one likes to feel helpless, especially when a loved one is suffering. Of course, anger and frustration also develop as a result of the annoying behaviors of people with mental illness.

The biggest danger with these feelings is that they may spill out in inappropriate ways. It is easy to get angry at your ill relative, or others in the family, for not doing things differently. As suggested in the Quick Reference Guide, Worksheet for Dealing with Your Anger and Frustration, you have many

WORKSHEET FOR DEALING WITH YOUR ANGER AND FRUSTRATION

Read over the following suggestions, filling in the blanks with ideas that apply to your situation.

I feel angry and frustrated when:

1. I am helpless to ease the suffering of someone I love.

2. Essential services are inadequate.

3. _____

4. _____

5. _____

I can avoid expressing these feelings in a manner that could be harmful to me or my relative by:

1. leaving the situation until I calm down

2. using a technique (fantasy, breathing, counting, etc.) to remain in the situation and handle it tactfully

3. _____

4. _____

5. _____

good reasons to feel angry. It is important that you do your best to identify exactly what it is about your particular situation that is so frustrating or infuriating. Find ways to deal with

Appropriate short-term outlets that are comfortable for me are:

1. telling a friend about it

2. exercising

3. yelling in my car

4. kicking a pillow at home

5. hitting a mattress with a tennis racket

6. _____

7. _____

I can channel my anger into long-term, constructive action by:

1. working with NAMI

2. writing legislators

3. doing volunteer work with people who have a mental illness

4. helping and supporting others in situations similar to my own

5. educating people about mental illness

6. _____

7. _____

the immediate situation that sparks the anger. Then try to find more constructive outlets for your anger. These might include directing your anger toward the illness rather than toward those afflicted or other family members, and toward the lack of services available. Only when enough people let their voices be heard will legislators give priority to allocating funds for the expansion of services for people with mental illness.

SMALL CHILDREN

Family members often wonder what, if anything, to say to small children about a relative with a mental illness and/or a substance-use problem. An ill person may have siblings, nieces, grandchildren, or others with whom they live or come in contact. It is important to find ways to talk with small children about the ill person and their behavior. There are ways to talk with children of any age in a manner that they can understand. Of course, you would give a different kind of explanation to a five-year-old than to a fifteen-year-old. With children of any age consider doing the following.

1. Acknowledge that the person has a problem with drugs or alcohol, is sick, has a mental illness, and what it is called.
2. Explain that the sickness makes him or her say and do things that he or she would not otherwise. Teenagers can be told and understand that it affects the person's thinking, feelings, behavior, and judgment.
3. Mention that the illness is not contagious. They need not worry about catching it.
4. Assure them it has nothing to do with them, or anything they did or said.

5. Reassure them that he or she still loves and cares about them even though the illness makes him or her do or say things that may make it seem otherwise.
6. Give specific instructions as to how to act around the person, including whether they should do or say things any differently than they would with others.

Children also need an opportunity to talk about what it is like for them to be around the person. If they are living with the person, children may have some anger, shame, embarrassment, confusion, disappointment, and so forth. If they have a chance to express these feelings to a compassionate adult within the family or to a professional outside the family, the illness will not take as great a toll as if they are left to suffer in secret. Families that are able to have ongoing discussions about the situation and hear and acknowledge the impact on everyone, tend to fare better than those that quietly bear the burden of the illness. Listening to and validating children's feelings go a long way toward helping them cope with difficult situations. You may not be able to make things all better, but you will be able to ameliorate some of the difficulties inherent in the situation.

Children should also be encouraged to continue with their usual activities and friendships as much as possible. It is important for them to be given permission to spend time and energy outside the family, with school, extracurricular activities, and friends. They may need to be reassured that it is not their responsibility to "fix" the ill person or other problems in the family that occur as a result of having an ill relative. It can also help to acknowledge the sadness you may feel that attending to the crises and illness sometimes detracts from the time, energy, and resources that would otherwise be devoted to them.

Balancing the Needs of Ill and Well Family Members

WE HAVE DISCUSSED THE special needs and experiences of people who suffer from a major mental illness, and the experiences and feelings that people who are close to a person with a mental illness will likely have. Now we will explore some of the problems that arise when caring people try to balance the needs of an ill relative with the needs of well family members.

Having a person with a mental illness in the family makes it difficult to consider each family member's unique needs when making decisions about how to allocate time, energy, and financial resources. You may often feel pulled in different directions or caught in the middle of a complex or impossible juggling act. The temptation may be to give your all to the ill person. This strategy will inevitably backfire. Rather, you must find a way to respect and consider everyone's needs, realizing that these will change as each person's situation changes. On some days or periods in your life you will be able to give more than at other times. In the beginning, you may be able to determine your limits only by trial and error. With experience you will learn what works best for everyone. The Quick Ref-

BALANCING TIME BETWEEN
ILL AND WELL FAMILY MEMBERS

To find the balance that is right for you, consider the following six questions:

1. How much time can you spend with your ill relative without resenting him or her (for example, two hours a day, one visit a week, one visit a month, one phone call a month)?

2. How much time do you need to spend with your ill relative in order to keep the relationship as good as possible in the long run?

3. How much time do other family members need and want? The fact that they are well makes them no less deserving.

4. How much nurturing do you need, via time spent alone and with well friends and family?

5. How enjoyable and valuable to you and your ill relative is the time you spend together? How does each of you feel after spending time together?

6. Are other well family members showing signs of stress (for example, physical symptoms, disturbances of sleep and eating habits, depression, and so forth)? Consider the price you or they may be paying for the lack of time and attention.

It is vital to you and the rest of your family that you not sacrifice all of your resources, time, energy, and money for your ill relative.

erence Guide entitled Balancing Time Between Ill and Well Family Members outlines some things to consider when trying to take everyone's needs into account.

TO BE OR NOT TO BE LIVING AT HOME

Perhaps the most painful and difficult decision families of people with mental illness face is whether to have their ill relative live with them. For some families, the decision is easy; their relatives need to be in a locked facility. Other people with mental illness are able and willing to live on their own, and need their family only for backup support. It is the millions in the middle who pose the biggest problem—one that could more easily be solved if the government would allocate money for a more extensive continuum of services for people with mental illness that would allow them to live in the community as independently as they can. Families could be involved with their ill relative, while retaining their own peaceful homes and separate lives. Unfortunately, since there are woefully fewer programs for people with mental illness than are needed in this country, families are often left to figure out how to deal with the situation by themselves.

As with so many challenges facing families and friends of people with mental illness, there are no clear and simple solutions. Each situation must be evaluated individually. The well-being of the ill person must be weighed against that of everyone else involved. Few people want to see their relative living on the streets or in a run-down hotel. However, having a seriously ill relative living at home is a major undertaking that puts an enormous strain on the rest of the family. It will inevitably have a significant impact on the relationships of everyone involved. Never underestimate the amount of energy it will require.

Some of the factors to weigh in making this decision are outlined in the Quick Reference Guide, Should My Relative Live at Home?

Remember that whatever choice you make can be revised over time as your circumstances and the course of the illness change. Periodically reevaluate your decision about where

SHOULD MY RELATIVE LIVE AT HOME?

There is no single answer to the question of whether your relative with a mental illness should live at home. The experience of most families and professionals suggests that people with mental illness generally seem to function at a higher level, and they and their families do better, when the ill person lives away from the home yet has support and contact with the family. Each family must carefully evaluate its own situation before making a decision. Having an ill relative live at home is more likely to work when:

1. The ill person functions at a fairly high level, without displaying many obvious symptoms.
2. The ill person has friends and activities outside the home.
3. The ill person is female.
4. No siblings live at home and so are not adversely affected by the presence of the ill relative.
5. The family has had family-skills training or is naturally calm, positive, respectful, and nonjudgmental toward the ill relative.

the ill person is to live and how much you are willing to relate to him or her.

Many people struggle to pull time and energy away from the ill person so there is some left over for the rest of the family and for themselves. For others, the struggle is to engage more often with the ill person even though this is painful and

6. The ill relative is agreeable to participating in some form of treatment and structured activity.

Having an ill relative live at home is not generally advised when:

1. The person's symptoms are so disruptive that the family cannot lead a reasonably normal life.
2. There are siblings living at home who feel adversely affected by living with the ill relative.
3. Family members become angry with the ill person, and frightened and critical of him or her.
4. The parents' marriage or relationship is strongly and negatively affected.
5. Family members become controlled by the ill person and are unable to engage in their usual activities and routines.
6. The ill relative has no outside activities or support system.
7. The family consists of a single parent living alone.
8. The ill person is actively abusing drugs or alcohol.

difficult. Completely disengaging from an ill relative is sometimes necessary, but never without its own pain. The Quick Reference Guide entitled Rules for Living at Home or Visiting is offered as a reminder that regardless of how extensive or

RULES FOR LIVING AT HOME OR VISITING

General guidelines for living at home or visiting:

1. Balance any special considerations your ill relative needs with the fact that all family members have rights.
2. Keep your expectations for your ill relative's behavior realistic.
3. Decisions regarding whether your relative should live at home or how long a visit will be should be negotiated with the person and based on:

   - his or her needs and wants
   - your needs and wants
   - his or her behavior
   - your tolerance for the person and his or her behavior

4. Have a few clear, basic house rules (for example, no violence, no smoking in bed, no radio or television after 11:00 P.M.).
5. Keep things as predictable as possible.

Visits:

1. Too short a visit is better than one that's too long. The most important thing is to communicate

minimal your contact with your ill relative is, you must pay attention to everyone's needs. It is better for you and your relative if you give only what you can give comfortably and freely, without overextending yourself.

warmth and love by your presence. If your relative is in a hospital or locked facility, this requires no more than one hour.

2. Tie the length of your relative's visit to overall or specific behavior.

3. Do not overprogram visits. Allow some quiet time amid the structured activity.

4. If your relative is home for a longer visit (one to two days), do not neglect the rest of your life during this time.

5. Encourage your relative to give input as to how the time will be spent.

6. Consider your own and other family members' preferences and needs as well as your ill relative's.

Living at home:

1. You and your relative need to get out of the house at different times and have separate activities.

2. Use consequences appropriate to the seriousness of violations.

3. Use natural consequences when possible. For example, if a privilege is abused, suspend that privilege.

4. Rules or consequences should change as your relative does.

MAKING ACTIVITIES AND HOLIDAYS ENJOYABLE

Many families and friends of people with mental illness are at a loss as to how to make activities with an ill loved one fun. Unfortunately, having fun is not always possible. Some people are too severely depressed or preoccupied with their internal worlds and delusions to be able to laugh or enjoy recreational activities. The best you can do for such people is

---

MAKING ACTIVITIES WITH THE ILL PERSON ENJOYABLE

If you are planning an outing with your relative:

1. Know what your relative can tolerate in terms of number of people, level of stimulation, travel time, and so on.

2. Know what you can tolerate in terms of what things embarrass you, how much time you can spend with your relative, and your level of anxiety about your relative.

3. Be willing to cancel this activity if your relative is doing poorly.

4. Go where people are more accepting of your relative's behavior and differences (for example, eat out at less formal restaurants).

5. Do not expect perfect performance, normal behavior, or anything beyond how the person usually behaves when slightly stressed.

If you are planning a get-together at home:

---

to provide enough contact and concern to let them know that you love and care about them, and to encourage them to comply with any treatments that help them.

Many others, however, can participate in and enjoy leisure-time activities if you devote a little special care and attention to planning the events. The Quick Reference Guide entitled Making Activities with the Ill Person Enjoyable outlines how to do this. The four most important rules to re-

1. Keep in mind your and your relative's respective levels of tolerance.
2. Often the best way to spend time together is to perform a task together. For larger family gatherings, try giving your relative a specific, task-oriented role (such as table setter, photographer, caretaker of the children, etc.).
3. Instruct other guests beforehand regarding your relative's needs, what to expect, and how to act.
4. Allow your relative to leave or take breaks whenever he or she needs to.

You can inoculate yourself from some upsets by:

1. beginning slowly and building levels of tolerance for spending recreational time together
2. avoiding surprises and discussing in advance what, to the best of your knowledge, the plan is
3. having a contingency plan if problems arise
4. keeping your expectations realistic
5. being flexible if things do not go as you had hoped. Never get attached to any one plan.

member: things will go better if your expectations are realistic; have a specific, prearranged plan; give your relative a concrete task or activity on which to focus; and accept the possibility that on any given day your relative may not feel well enough to follow through on a prearranged activity.

In planning a visit or outing, take into account your relative's present level of functioning and interests. If he or she has recently come out of the hospital, going to a baseball game may overwhelm him or her because of the crowd, even if your relative is a sports buff. It is good to discuss in advance the kinds of activities your relative is currently comfortable with.

It is also important to keep in mind the kinds of activities you are comfortable with. Let's say your relative wants to go to a fancy restaurant but you know that he or she often forgets to shower, tends to talk in a loud voice, is a little bizarre, and embarrasses you in quiet restaurants. If you take your relative to the place of his or her choice, you are likely to have an awful time. You would be much better off going to a noisy family-style restaurant, or suggesting a picnic in the park or a trip to the local zoo. Your needs are as important as your relative's, so consider both. This takes some creativity, but is well worth the effort.

Most people with a mental illness are uncomfortable with unstructured social time during which there are no activities to focus on and everyone is sitting around making small talk. Such situations tend to highlight what is lacking or problematic in their lives. After a few minutes no one is sure what to talk about and everyone's level of anxiety begins to rise. You would do far better to find some common interest on which to focus: a game, a movie, a sports event, a simple walk, or anything else that takes the focus and pressure off the person's having to talk about his or her life or to fill up the silence.

The length of time you spend together is less important

than the quality of the visit. It usually works better for everyone involved if visits are kept short. Nothing is accomplished in the extra time; one or the other of you will probably just get uncomfortable. Your relative needs to know that you are there and that you care about him or her. This can be achieved quite effectively with a regular phone call or a brief visit.

Holidays

Holidays in particular are difficult for many families with a member who has a mental illness. We often have expectations that everyone will be happy, feel good, and have a great time at holiday get-togethers. These expectations are unrealistic and consequently can cause more depression and despair than usual for people with a mental illness and their loved ones. There are, however, several things you can do to counteract this.

One important guideline is to be honest with yourself and your loved one about how he or she, and you, are feeling. For instance, if your relative knows it is okay to tell you that he or she is not looking forward to seeing all the cousins at Christmas, doesn't have enough money to buy any presents, hates to go shopping anyway, and is not sure he or she will show up for the big holiday celebration, you are way ahead of the game. If the person believes he or she has to pretend to feel great about it all, things will probably go badly. The person will likely feel more stressed, and his or her symptoms could easily become more severe.

If you can understand and accept that birthdays, anniversaries, and the holiday season are likely to be somewhat painful times, your relationship with your ill relative will be greatly improved. If you can let the person know that you love him or her and will be delighted if he or she attends the holiday activities, but will also understand if he or she feels too uncomfortable to do so, your relationship will not be scarred by the stress of the holidays.

Some families prefer to alter their way of celebrating so that the ill person will feel more comfortable. This may mean reducing the number of people involved in a get-together, the length of the event, and its degree of formality, and not serv-

HANDLING THE HOLIDAYS

Holidays tend to be especially stressful for people with a mental illness because:

1. There are often implied, if not explicit, expectations of certain types of behavior (e.g., exchanging of gifts), feelings (happiness), and so on that they may not be able to live up to.
2. Large groups can be overstimulating and confusing.
3. Holidays can be painful reminders of times past when things were better, thus highlighting present disabilities.
4. Family get-togethers can raise the issue of what the ill person is to tell people about his or her life, illness, and so forth.
5. Holidays lend themselves to ill people comparing themselves unfavorably to other (perhaps younger), higher-functioning or more accomplished relatives.

You can help your relative reduce the stress by:

ing alcohol. Other families decide to have several events—a smaller one with the ill person and a larger one without him or her. Consider any creative solution that works for your family. There is no right or wrong with these questions. You would do well to review the Quick Reference Guide, Handling the Holidays, before you plan any major festivities.

1. discussing plans in advance
2. acknowledging any mixed feelings he or she may have. Do not make assumptions about how he or she will feel or act.
3. keeping expectations realistic, especially regarding whether your relative can tolerate a gathering, for how long, and what kind of participation he or she is capable of
4. respecting and supporting your relative's choices and decisions regarding whether he or she is comfortable participating and in what way
5. accepting your and your relative's limits
6. helping your relative figure out how to handle some of the stress (e.g., how the person might answer questions, what task he or she might like to focus on, how long to stay, places to go to take breaks), if he or she is willing and able to discuss the event and his or her feelings. It may be important to acknowledge all family members' needs, preferences, and limits before a workable solution can be reached.

FAMILY PROBLEM-SOLVING
AND DECISION MAKING

All families and groups function better if they have agreements about how decisions will be made and problems solved. Without clarity in these areas, life becomes more stressful and relationships tend to deteriorate. Since problems, decisions, and stress increase when mental illness is involved, it is especially important to develop constructive methods of decision making and problem-solving in these situations.

The Quick Reference Guide entitled Family Problem-Solving outlines a technique that has been helpful for many families. You may choose to follow it exactly, or you may decide to modify it in a way that better suits your family. What is important is that you evolve an effective way to handle problems that does not add unnecessary stress to your life. Just as important as the problem-solving technique you adopt is the mechanism by which everyone involved becomes familiar and reasonably comfortable with the technique. This will take time and practice. If everyone can agree on the fact that there is a problem and on the method of approaching it, you are well on your way to a solution. You may want to establish a ground rule that a problem exists if someone feels that it does.

Defining the problem can go a long way toward bringing out what is upsetting people. Often people see things from their own different and somewhat limited perspective. For example, one person may feel that another is always ignoring him or her. It may be that only when this problem is clearly stated will the other person feel free to say that he or she is feeling constantly criticized. It is wise to consider both points of view as expressing problems and to begin to look for solutions that will leave both people feeling heard and considered.

Generating as many solutions as possible is the next important step. Encourage everyone to express whatever ideas come to mind. Do not at this point limit yourselves to realistic, logical solutions. You want to encourage everyone to come up with as many different ways of dealing with the problem as possible. You may be surprised at the realistic solutions that emerge from even the most absurd ones.

FAMILY PROBLEM-SOLVING

Step 1. Arrange a family meeting. Include as many family members as possible.

Step 2. Define the problem. Talk about it. Listen carefully, ask questions, and get everyone's opinion. Then write down exactly what the problem is.

Step 3. List all possible solutions. Write down all ideas, even bad ones. Get everybody to come up with at least one possible solution.

Step 4. Discuss each possible solution. Go down the list and discuss the advantages and disadvantages of each possible solution.

Step 5. Choose the best solution or combination of solutions.

Step 6. Plan how to carry out the best solution. Come up with a step-by-step procedure.

Step 7. Revise the solution if necessary. Do not be afraid to drop a solution that does not work and start again.

Although you may not want to go through every step with every problem, remember that the more organized your approach to problem-solving is, the better your chances of success.

Next, make a clear distinction between the brainstorming process and the next step—discussing each idea from a rational viewpoint. Keep as positive an attitude as possible throughout. Remember, the process of dealing with problems is, in the long run, more important than the solution to any one problem. You want to encourage everyone to participate, and to praise people for whatever level of involvement they are capable of. The person with a mental illness may not always come up with the most practical solutions, but may think of more creative or interesting ones than anyone else. Try to make the overall experience as enjoyable and as much of a team effort as possible.

In selecting the best alternative or combination of ideas, you need to begin to be specific about how the solution will be implemented: exactly who will do what, where, when, and how. Leave as little to the imagination as possible.

Once you decide on a solution, always give it a trial run. It works well to establish, in advance, a time to evaluate the solution. Everyone should stay open to the possibility of revising or modifying the solution as experience dictates. It is impossible to think of all eventualities in advance. The more you can encourage everyone to look at problems as a team, making a team response and evaluation, the more smoothly your lives will run.

If you still cannot agree on a solution or if you do not have time to go through the process, you nevertheless need to have some understanding about how decisions will be made. The Quick Reference Guide, What to Do When You Can't Agree on What to Do, underscores the fact that you will have disagreements about what to do and that you will need to have ways of resolving these differences.

Patterns in your disputes are likely to emerge over time. Try to be as patient with yourself and the rest of your family as you can. Consider the likelihood that all viewpoints have some validity. Individual strengths and weaknesses will emerge over time. For example, one family member may be more comfortable at handling telephone calls, while another is adept at dealing with crises. Without condemning anyone, try to make the best use of everyone's skills.

WHAT TO DO WHEN YOU CAN'T AGREE ON WHAT TO DO

You must decide in advance what decision-making process works best for your family. The possibilities include democracy (one person, one vote); consensus and compromise; and one authority who solicits input from others involved.

Remember that it is natural for families to have differences of opinion regarding such issues as how much your ill relative should be asked to do for himself or herself, where your relative should live, how to get your relative to follow through on requests or agreements, how serious a particular situation is, how to handle a crisis, and so on.

In attempting to resolve differences, remember that there is no right or wrong. Think about what might work best for your relative and your family.

Discuss with the family what you imagine to be the worst-case scenario for each alternative, based on past experiences.

Think of options you have tried that did not work well as sources of useful information. You are like a researcher; you cannot have all the answers until every effort has been made.

PROBLEM-SOLVING BETWEEN PARENT AND CHILD

A particular kind of tension often exists between the parent of a person with a mental illness and the sibling of the ill person. Many parents and children have struggled long and hard with the differing amounts of involvement that each wanted with the ill person. While parents often have strong feelings about their children's lack of involvement with an ill sibling,

WHAT PARENTS CAN AND CANNOT DO FOR SIBLINGS

Parents can:

- be aware that all family members are profoundly affected.
- be aware of the coping stance that siblings may adopt—for example, estrangement or enmeshment.
- talk about their feelings and encourage siblings to do the same.
- learn about the illness and thereby lower family anxiety.
- avoid making the ill member the axis around which the family revolves. This is as detrimental to the ill person as it is to other family members.
- seek to improve the mental-health system so that more after-care options are available following hospitalization.
- read articles and books on sibling relationships to have a better understanding of the sibling expe-

children may have equally strong feelings about their parent's extensive involvement with that person.

The Sibling and Adult Children Network, a former subgroup of NAMI, has put a good deal of effort into bridging the gap that often exists between parents and well children. The Quick Reference Guide entitled What Parents Can and Cannot Do for Siblings is largely based on the efforts of this group. The guidelines given here are applicable to differences

rience, and provide such resources to siblings if they are interested.

Parents cannot:

- take away the fact that mental illness has an impact on other siblings.
- lessen the impact by not talking about it.
- shield siblings from their own feelings about it.
- determine the coping style individual siblings may adopt.
- experience the grieving process for siblings. Everyone must go through this process, which usually includes denial, depression, anger, and finally, acceptance, in his or her own way, at his or her own pace.
- make siblings seek help during the denial stage.
- expect siblings not to experience a variety of negative emotions such as guilt, fear, grief, resentment, and jealousy.

among other family members as well, and underscore the painful limitations in our ability to fix situations with which we all must struggle.

Some siblings have found writings on co-dependency useful. Also, *Hidden Victims,* written specifically for siblings and adult children of people with mental illness by Julie Johnson, and *Troubled Journey: Coming to Terms with the Mental Illness of a Sibling or Parent,* by Diane Marsh and Rex Dickens, contain material that is relevant not only to siblings but to other family members as well. Many parents find that participation in twelve-step programs such as CoDA (Co-dependents Anonymous) and Al-Anon is quite helpful to them.

KEEPING THE FAMILY STRONG

Every family will experience conflict as it struggles to balance the needs of a seriously disabled member with the needs of its other members. Disagreements are unavoidable, given the degree of stress and uncertainty that mental illness brings. Remember, the best you can do is to agree on ways to handle problems when they arise, and then agree that sometimes you will disagree on the best way to proceed.

The way to keep the family strong is to consider everyone's preferences and limitations when making decisions. Whether you are deciding how to spend a few hours together on Sunday or where your ill relative should live, pay careful attention to the needs of all involved and strive to find a balance that works reasonably well for everyone concerned. Nobody can get all of what he or she wants all the time. Everyone has to make compromises and adjustments to maintain relationships; when mental illness is part of the equation, the adjustments and compromises will likely be magnified.

Working with
Mental-Health Professionals
and Choosing Facilities

*F*INDING YOUR WAY THROUGH the maze of the mental-health system is no simple feat. Families often find that their interactions with professionals and facilities range from confusing and frustrating to infuriating and insulting. In order to understand why the situation is so difficult, it is important to know some of the history of the system, how and when various forms of treatment were developed, and the impact on the system of various legal, political, and economic forces.

A BRIEF HISTORY OF
THE MENTAL-HEALTH SYSTEM

The United States does not have a well-thought-out system of services for its citizens with mental illness. For most of the last century, people with mental illness were kept in large institutions, out of sight and out of mind. Then in the 1950s antipsychotic medications were discovered, and the level of functioning for a significant number of people was increased. This opened up the possibility of people with mental illness living with a much lower level of care than institutions provided.

In the 1960s, during the Kennedy administration, a plan was developed to close institutions and create a more humane system of caring for people with mental illness in homelike settings in the community. Unfortunately, more than forty years later, only about half of that noble plan has been implemented: many institutions have been closed. And although we have learned how to care for people with mental illness in the community through supported-housing, vocational, case-management, and socialization programs, few of these programs exist, and the funds to create more have not been allocated.

This unfortunate situation is further complicated by laws governing parents' rights. In the mid twentieth century, it was not terribly difficult to have someone committed to a mental hospital. Many people fell victim to the laws that permitted this. Patients, ex-patients, and their advocates eventually banded together to get the laws changed. They succeeded—but, as is so often the case, the unjust laws were replaced with laws so extreme that they created a new set of problems.

The good news is that patients' rights are now well protected. The bad news is that it is now almost impossible to get people treated against their will. There may be clear evidence that they are much happier and that their lives work much better when they are on medication. There may be a clear indication that a psychotic episode is under way and that medication or a brief hospitalization could cut short the severity and length of the episode. None of this may be sufficient to require treatment for a person with mental illness. In most states, unless there is a clear and present danger to oneself or others, a person has the right to refuse treatment. This can frustrate both mental-health workers and families. Legislation to change these laws is now under consideration.

The psychological theories of mental illness that were popular in the 1950s and 1960s have also had a lingering impact on families and friends of people with mental illness. Theorists such as Gregory Bateson, Jay Haley, Don Jackson, and John Weakland tended to blame families—especially mothers—for causing the problems. Many mental-health professionals were taught that families caused the disorders, and, consequently, they treated families with disdain. Many families were deeply wounded by such misguided professionals.

The tide has definitely turned. Now most professionals, especially those who work directly with people with severe mental illness, believe that these illnesses are biological and are not caused by the family environment. As a result, they now tend to treat families with respect, compassion, and openness. They are more willing to work with families as allies in dealing with a tragic illness (albeit within the framework of a grossly underfunded and inadequate system).

For a discussion of the history, politics, and economics of the mental-health system in the United States, I recommend *Madness in the Streets: How Psychiatry and the Law Abandoned the Mentally Ill,* by Rael Isaac and Virginia Armat. Douglas Polcin's article, "Administrative Planning in Community Mental Health," which appeared in the *Community Mental Health Journal,* is also very informative.

WHO'S WHO ON THE TEAM

The most advanced approach to working with people with a severe mental illness involves a team approach, consisting of the consumer, family, and several professionals with varying specialties, backgrounds, and training. The professionals include:

The psychiatrist. Previously assumed to be the team leader, this person has an M.D., indicating that he or she has completed medical school and has specialized in psychiatry (as opposed to pediatrics, internal medicine, or any one of numerous other specialties). Only M.D.s can prescribe medication. Not all psychiatrists have much experience or training in working with adults who have a serious mental illness.

The psychologist. This person has six to eight years of postgraduate training. Psychologists are also called *doctor,* but that's because they have received a doctor of philosophy (Ph.D.). Psychologists usually work in a consulting role or give psychological tests. They cannot prescribe medication, but in many programs they serve a function similar to that of a psychiatrist.

The social worker. Social workers usually have at least two years of postgraduate training, and a master's degree in social work (M.S.W.). Most states have a related degree and license for marriage and family therapists (M.F.T.s).

All of the professionals mentioned above may have a private practice in which they offer psychotherapy, for which they accept various forms of medical insurance. However, you are cautioned to check into these providers, as the training they receive may or may not include experience with people with serious mental illnesses. There are efforts currently under way to include information about mental illnesses in all training programs, but this step has not yet been taken in many colleges and universities.

Numerous other professionals work with people who have a serious mental illness as part of multidisciplinary treatment teams. They may be employed as staff members in hospitals, residential programs, day treatment centers, and so on. They usually have at least two years of college-level training, and include occupational therapists (O.T.s), recreational thera-

pists (R.T.s), psychiatric nurses (R.N.s), psychiatric techni-
cians (P.T.s), and counselors. Counselors usually have experience working with people with mental illness and/or a
bachelor's or associate (two years of college) degree in psychology, counseling, or a related field.

With other illnesses, a doctor oversees the overall course
of treatment. This is not often the case with a mental illness.
The doctor involved may be affiliated with a hospital, but he
or she may not be able or willing to follow the course of the
illness after the patient has been released from the hospital.

One excellent alternative method, in practice in many areas, is to have a case manager oversee the care once it becomes
clear that a person will need ongoing assistance. Case managers may be professionals with a bachelor's or master's degree in social work, psychology, counseling, or a related field,
or paraprofessionals with on-the-job training in this kind of
work. They coordinate services with ill people as they move
from one program or service to another, and help with the
transitions. The staff supporting those programs may work
with the ill people to help them meet their vocational, social,
and practical needs (housing, money, structured activities, and
so forth). If a person is able to live independently, it may be the
case manager who provides assistance in meeting basic needs,
as well as in locating health professionals such as therapists,
doctors, and dentists, in obtaining medication and financial
assistance, and in gaining access to other resources that will
allow the person to remain stable in the community and minimize the need for hospitalizations or more intensive care.

The intensive case-management programs that have been
established in various parts of the country have had impressive
success. A well-trained, concerned case manager can make a
significant difference in the life of a person with a serious mental illness, dramatically improving the person's quality of life
and keeping crises and hospitalizations to a minimum.

THE DIVISION OF RESPONSIBILITY IN YOUR RELATIVE'S LIFE AND TREATMENT

The ill relative:

- assumes as much responsibility as possible for his or her own life and behavior
- does his or her best to live a satisfying life
- sets goals and works with service providers and family to achieve them

The family:

- offers love and an ongoing, supportive relationship within realistic limits
- encourages the relative to participate in and cooperate with treatment and services
- finds out how it can support the treatment
- does everything it can to protect the relative from serious danger
- educates its members about the illness and the mental-health system

The doctor or therapist:

- provides an ongoing, long-term therapeutic relationship
- provides a diagnosis, prognosis, and overview of the course of the illness
- prescribes and monitors medication

- provides education about the medication
- arranges for hospitalizations when necessary

The case manager:

- assists the ill person in meeting essential needs and remaining stable in the community
- makes referrals to various treatment programs and community resources and assists in transitions from one program or service to another
- supplies historical information to service providers and provides continuity as the ill person moves through the mental-health system and community resources
- provides crisis intervention when other treatment staff are not involved

The treatment-program staff provides a therapeutic environment that may include:

- ongoing support, therapeutic relationships, and assistance with establishing realistic goals and plans
- education, training, or counseling in areas such as life skills, vocational goals, interpersonal skills, coping with symptoms, and acceptance of limitations
- crisis intervention
- documentation of the course of treatment and progress made
- supervision of medication

However, things rarely work this smoothly. There is currently a shortage of case-management services, and many people with mental illness refuse to go to the hospital or emergency psychiatric services in the first place. As a result many people suffer without the treatment that could relieve their pain. Families, friends, doctors, therapists, and treatment staff alike are unable to intervene, and so watch helplessly as people they care about deteriorate. It is unfortunate that so often a family's anger gets turned against the staff of hospitals or programs for not doing more to make their relative well. The staff would probably like nothing better than to be able to do just that. However, they are usually working in a program that is underfunded, and they are understaffed, overworked, and underpaid. They share the same frustration and outrage that families feel about how inadequate the available services are.

When people have a serious mental illness and, due to the illness, are a danger to themselves or others or are unable to provide for their own basic needs for food, clothing, and shelter, someone else may be given legal authority to meet the person's needs and to make certain decisions about the person's life and, sometimes, property. This legal structure is called a *guardianship* or *conservatorship*. The person appointed is called a *conservator* or *guardian*. The conservator/guardian may be a county employee or a family member; the decision is made at a court hearing.

The conservator may make decisions about where a person will live, whether or not he or she must be in a hospital or treatment program, who will manage the person's money and, in some states, whether the person may travel, drive, or enter into contractual agreements. Only by means of a guardianship or conservatorship can someone be treated involuntarily for any length of time. To find out the specifics of how guardianships work in your state, contact your local NAMI or public guardian's office.

There are advantages and disadvantages to having a conservator for someone unable to care for himself or herself. Whether a family member should take on the job of being a relative's conservator is almost as weighty a question as whether an ill relative should live at home. It warrants the same kind of careful examination of your individual situation.

The Quick Reference Guide entitled The Division of Responsibility in Your Relative's Life and Treatment summarizes the role that everyone involved with a person who has a mental illness plays in the best-designed system of services. Of course, most systems are far less than ideal. Therefore, one or another of the key players often has to assume a job that should be performed by someone else. Frequently there are no case managers available because of lack of government funding. A family member, program staff member, or doctor may wind up doing all or part of the job. Or the role may be left unfilled, causing services and treatment to occur in a chaotic, disorganized way. This guide is offered so that you can be aware of the kind of system we are working toward and to help you evaluate the level of services available in your community.

Remember that no one, not even the most loving, educated family or the most expert professional, can assume full responsibility for another adult's life or well-being.

Ideally, all members of the treatment team are periodically in contact with one another to coordinate the care your relative is receiving. They may do so by telephone or at periodic treatment-planning conferences. The more progressive programs will invite family members to participate in some or all of these meetings. What is likely to happen there is described in the Quick Reference Guide entitled Planning Conferences. It

PLANNING CONFERENCES

Why, when, and where do planning conferences occur?
The purpose of these meetings is for all those involved
with the treatment or life of a client to:

1. share current and historical information regarding
   the client

2. generate a consistent plan and approach in working with the client

Conferences are ideally scheduled once every few
months or when significant changes are happening in a
person's life or situation, and are held at the time and
place most convenient for all involved. They usually last
about one hour at most.

Who usually attends planning conferences?

1. the treating M.D. or therapist

2. staff representatives from the programs the client
   is involved in—for example, residential, day, or
   vocational programs; hospital or psychiatric emergency services

3. the case manager

The client and family members are ideally invited to
the entire meeting or a portion of it.

What usually happens during a conference?

1. Information is exchanged. Each person reviews
   the client's progress (or lack thereof) since the last
   conference or since he or she began working with
   the client. In addition, people may need to acquaint

one another with the services they or their programs offer, relevant procedures, and so forth.

2. Each person's understanding of the client's dynamics, strengths, problems, and goals is identified.

3. When the client appears, he or she will usually be asked for his or her views regarding number 2 above and be informed of the concerns and recommendations of the team.

4. A plan is discussed and agreed upon that addresses:

   - which areas most need attention and how team members will work with the client toward identified goals

   - any changes that need to occur and how they will be implemented, such as placement, medication, and so forth

   - when the next conference will occur

How can family members prepare for and contribute to planning conferences?

1. Bring with you any important historical information that you think may not be known to those attending.

2. Present concise descriptions of recent behavior, especially any changes you have observed in your relative.

3. Prepare or make brief statements regarding:

   - concerns you have about your relative and/or the current treatment

   - recommendations about how these or other concerns may best be addressed

is well worth reviewing this guide before you attend a conference, especially if you have never been to one before.

DEALING WITH MENTAL-HEALTH WORKERS

The relationship you establish with the treatment professionals involved with your relative is important. Giving some thought to how you deal with them can have a significant impact on the way in which they respond to you. The basics to keep in mind are summarized in the Quick Reference Guide

DEALING WITH MENTAL-HEALTH PROFESSIONALS AND FACILITIES

To enhance your relationships with professionals and service providers:

1. Be courteous. Courtesy is to your advantage as a consumer and as an advocate for your relative.
2. Provide information.
3. Be respectful of their time.
4. Ask how you can be involved in a supportive way.
5. Request meetings, with or without your relative present, when you feel the need. In addition, you may ask for a diagnosis, treatment plan, medication information, and prognosis (though your relative's consent may be required).

entitled Dealing with Mental-Health Professionals and Facilities. These suggestions may seem obvious, but in the middle of a crisis or difficult situation they are often forgotten.

Remember, don't base your evaluation of the value of a facility on one interaction. There are wide variations in competence and sensitivity within all programs. Furthermore, you have more in common with the staff than you may think. They want what is best for your relative, even though you may not agree with them on what that is. They are just as frustrated, angered, and saddened by the mental-health situation in this country as you are. By viewing them as allies,

6. Expect to be treated respectfully and with consideration.

7. Keep in mind the frustrations and constraints professionals face, such as:

- their inability to help patients who will not accept treatment

- the stigma, prejudice, and ignorance regarding mental illness that they and their clients face

- the desire of families for unrealistic results (cures)

- patients who do not improve because of our limited knowledge regarding the treatment of people with mental illness

- the lack of adequate funding for programs, staff, and patients' essential needs

- laws regarding confidentiality

TREATMENT SETTINGS AND SERVICES

RESIDENTIAL PROGRAMS (client lives at the facility)

Hospitals. Twenty-four-hour supervision; patients have minimal responsibilities for meeting their own basic needs. May be long-term-care facilities for the chronically ill (usually state hospitals) or short-term acute-care units run privately or by cities or counties. May be locked or unlocked.

Skilled nursing facilities. Twenty-four-hour supervision; patients have minimal responsibilities for basic needs. Usually provide long-term care. Locked.

Halfway houses and residential treatment programs. Usually time limited.

Board and care. Open, small, homelike environments or larger boarding homes where a house parent, owner, or operator makes sure that basic needs are met. Requires some level of self-care and symptom control.

Assisted independent living or supported housing programs. Various arrangements that involve renting individually or cooperatively run apartments or houses. Requires a high level of responsibility and self-care. Staff may be available to help things run smoothly, but are not on the premises twenty-four hours a day. Services may be provided by one agency or by an "integrated service team." This is a collaboration of agencies each providing specialized services, such as nursing and substance-abuse or mental-health counseling.

OUTPATIENT SERVICES (client lives elsewhere)

Clinics. May be run privately or run by counties or cities; may be called community mental-health centers. May offer individual, group, and family therapy, and monitoring of medication.

Case-management services. May be publicly or privately run. Assist and support people to maintain within the community.

Day treatment programs. Offer therapeutic activities, groups, and outings for a wide range of clients.

Vocational programs. Provide preparation for, counseling for, and coaching before and during employment in the community. Some provide jobs within the program and sheltered workshops.

Socialization programs. Sometimes called creative living centers or clubhouse-model programs. May be run by consumers or professionals. Offer recreational activities, self-help groups, and a varying range of other activities.

Emergency services. These include psychiatric emergency units (often part of the county hospital), emergency food and housing services, suicide prevention hotlines, and the police department.

Social services. Most counties and cities have a department, which may or may not offer many services to people with mental illness.

Legal services. Patients'-rights advocates, public defenders, the Legal Aid Society, the public guardian's office, and private attorneys can offer legal advice.

your exchanges with them will probably be much more satisfying. By joining forces we can make the system work to its
potential. Venting your anger and frustration at them only
makes their jobs harder and encourages them to be less open
to and supportive of you.

Additionally, keep in mind that you are likely to get more
detailed and informative responses from professionals by
showing that you know something about the illness, treat-

RESIDENTIAL TREATMENT PROGRAMS

Services provided:

1. twenty-four-hour staff coverage. Most houses are
   staffed by people genuinely interested in and
   trained to work with people with mental illness.
   Their level of education varies from a few years of
   college to a Ph.D.

2. a homelike environment in a community setting

3. assistance organizing such household functions
   as shopping, cooking, and cleaning

4. individual counseling, which may focus on personal problems, acceptance of the illness, hygiene, money management, and vocational or
   educational interests

5. crisis intervention

6. treatment planning and coordination in conjunction with a doctor, case manager, and others involved

7. supervision of medications

ments, and the mental-health system. Don't pretend to be an expert; just ask informed questions. Questions like "How is he, Doc?" are not as effective as queries such as "Do you think this is an isolated episode or part of a long-term illness like schizophrenia or bipolar disorder?" or "Do you have a working diagnosis? What do you think the prognosis is?" or "How long a hospitalization do you anticipate that this will be? Is there a discharge date set yet?" or "Do the medications

8. opportunities for social interaction with peers, which affords a chance to learn and practice social skills
9. structured activities

Services not provided:

1. constant individual attention
2. supervision while residents are off the premises
3. the safety and security of a locked facility
4. complete control over residents' actions and behavior. For example, a residential program cannot assure that clients will take their medication or see their doctor.
5. a guarantee of success
6. private rooms (in most cases)

Each program has certain minimal requirements to which the residents must adhere in order to remain in good standing. These usually include doing chores, as well as abstaining from violence and the use of illegal drugs.

seem to be helping him very much?" or "How likely is it that she will be able to take care of herself after being released from the hospital?" or "Do you think he will need a rehabilitation program after discharge?" or "What kind of approach seems to work best in your dealing with her?"

Throughout this book, I have emphasized how important it is to keep your expectations realistic both for yourself and for your ill relative. The same is true of your expectations for mental-health professionals and treatment programs or facilities. These people and programs are limited in the services they can provide, and the illnesses themselves limit how effective they can be. While it is reasonable to hope and expect that your relative's participation in a program will help reduce his or her symptoms, such a program cannot make the symptoms go away entirely. Familiarizing yourself with the specific services available in your area is of great importance. The two Quick Reference Guides—entitled Treatment Settings and Services and Residential Treatment Programs—describe some of the kinds of services available in this country.

Most programs work to help people learn to accept their limitations and to teach them basic living and interpersonal skills. While some people need to relearn previously known skills, others need to learn skills that they never had owing to the onset of the illness at an early age. They may learn how to better recognize and manage stress and the symptoms they experience when crises develop. A good program also teaches people how to set realistic goals for themselves and how to formulate the small steps they can take to achieve their goals. One common outcome of participating in a program is that clients develop a social support system. They meet people with whom they have much in common and with whom they subsequently become friends.

A crucial role for families is to encourage their loved one to participate in and cooperate with whatever program he or she is involved in. Your support can help your relative succeed in a program. Giving him or her mixed messages about the program or bad-mouthing the staff can undermine the chances for success. Think of you and the program staff as two sets of parents. If both sets of parents work together, life goes far more smoothly than if one set (you) becomes competitive or acts in open conflict with the other (staff). Just as children tend to try to pit one parent against another to avoid doing what they need to do, people in treatment programs may try to get parents or friends to argue with program staff. You are strongly advised to check with staff before getting too upset about the complaint or report you hear from your relative. It is hard to know what really happened without hearing both sides and determining the context in which an event occurred. Remember, people with mental illness tend to be confused and to distort reality, even with the best of intentions.

For example, Ruth, a woman in a residential treatment program, called her parents to say they should come and pick her up because her counselor said that she could leave the program and live on her own. Upon investigation the parents found out that their daughter had a conversation that actually went something like this:

RUTH:	I hate this place. I hate being told to do my chores and dealing with all these crazy people. I want to leave and get my own apartment.
COUNSELOR:	I'm not sure you are ready to do that just yet. You seem to be angry with the cleaning-committee person who just told you to make your bed.
RUTH:	(shouting): I don't have to make my bed if I don't want to. I could just get my own place and do whatever I want and

you can't stop me. I signed myself into
this place and I could sign myself out,
couldn't I?

COUNSELOR: Yes, you could, but I don't think it
would be a very good idea for you to do
that right now. Why don't you sit down
for a while until you feel calm? Then we
can discuss it further.

RUTH: Fine, but I want to talk to my family
first. I'm going to call them right now.

While what Ruth told her parents was literally correct, it
was not at all what the counselor had advised her to do. Yet
her parents would have had no way of knowing this without
talking to the counselor.

This is not to say that all complaints or concerns from a
relative are unfounded and should be ignored. There may be
inappropriate or improper things going on that you need to
know about. Investigate the complaint and inform the program director or other authority if needed. Just make sure
your information is as accurate as possible.

CONFIDENTIALITY

The issue of confidentiality is often a sticky one between families and professionals. It is best to have your relative sign a
paper indicating that he or she gives permission for a particular person or facility to release information to you about his
or her treatment, diagnosis, and prognosis. You can write out
your own release form or make a copy of the sample Authorization for Release of Confidential Information provided
here. When you obtain such a letter, it relieves professionals
of having to worry about the legalities involved in releasing
confidential information.

AUTHORIZATION FOR RELEASE OF
CONFIDENTIAL INFORMATION

I, _____, hereby give permission for
   (print patient's name)

_____ to release information
   (doctor, therapist, or facility)

to _____ my _____,
   (print your name)   (relationship to patient)

about my condition and treatment.

This authorization is valid indefinitely ❏ (check box
if no termination date) or until _____.

                              (termination date)

_____   _____
(patient's signature)   (date)

Of course, your relative may not be willing to cooperate. In such a case the staff is bound by law to maintain confidentiality. There are, however, ways the professionals involved can still give you information, if they are so inclined, such as by talking in generalities or with some degree of vagueness. For instance, a doctor who has just seen your son may tell you that often people who have these kinds of illnesses also have problems with drugs like LSD. He or she may be trying to give you important information without violating a confidence told to him or her by your son.

On the other hand, the relationship between the therapist and patient must also be respected. If a person is paranoid or mistrustful, learning that his or her therapist has been talking to family members can mar their relationship. There are ways to handle this, if the professional believes it is important for the lines of communication to be open. Again, getting written consent in advance from your relative will increase the likelihood that professionals will share information with you. Try to obtain the consent when you and your relative are calm and on good terms.

There is also nothing wrong with calling a hospital or treatment program and asking for a general progress report. Again, it helps if you can tell the facility that you have a written release of information from your relative. Do not be hesitant to call if the facility has not called you. It may be a busy place whose staff has not yet had a chance to call you. It also may have no way of knowing that you exist. You do not want to nag the facility, but you do want the staff to know that you are concerned and want to be updated periodically so that you can be available to help with the treatment plan.

KEEPING A TREATMENT RECORD

In the best of all worlds, there would be one master treatment record kept for each person with a mental illness. It would immediately be made available to all treatment personnel who see the person. But in this far-from-perfect world such a record most often does not exist. Even when some approximation of it does exist, it is not always readily available. It takes time for one facility to transfer records to another.

Therefore, another crucial function for families is to keep such a record. I strongly urge you to do so. Of course, you

KEEPING A TREATMENT RECORD OF YOUR OWN

Include the following information in your record:

1. Level of functioning prior to becoming ill. Highest level of school completed, work experience, level of basic life skills (cooking, cleaning, money management, independent-living experience), social skills and relationships with peers, strengths and significant achievements.

2. Symptoms. When they began, what they are, most effective ways of dealing with them, dates of more severe episodes.

3. Treatment. Dates of the first psychiatric hospitalization or treatment. How long it lasted. The diagnosis. How much improvement there was afterward. What psychiatric medication has been tried, when, how effective it was, and how serious the side effects were. Include similar information for any subsequent hospitalizations or involvement with treatment programs.

4. Level of functioning between hospitalizations or involvements in treatment programs.

5. Names, addresses, and phone numbers of all doctors, therapists, and service providers involved with the person.

6. Medical-insurance coverage and policy number.

may not be privy to each and every stop your relative makes in a hospital or program. But if you keep the best record you can and make it available each time your relative is admitted to a new program or starts working with a new therapist or ongoing service provider, you will be offering invaluable information. (Note that the staff may or may not have the ability to acknowledge this to you.)

The record need not be lengthy or extremely detailed; what you want to offer is an overview. The Quick Reference Guide, Keeping a Treatment Record of Your Own, outlines what should be included. Such a record can also be helpful in justifying the need for treatment or a conservatorship.

WORKING TOGETHER

Few programs, or even hospitals, for people with a mental illness have well-developed statements of philosophy or guidelines for the staff's contact with families. Even fewer have thought about what the role of family members could be if we all worked together toward the same goal.

Let us assume that we all want people with mental illness to function as well as they can and to have the best relationship possible with their families. This could most likely be achieved if programs and hospitals interacted with families in the following way:

1. During the admission procedure or preadmission screening (if one exists), prospective patients/clients would whenever possible be advised of the program's policy and philosophy of maintaining contact with families.
2. Admission agreements would reflect this philosophy.

3. Families would be contacted when a relative was admitted. Information about the program and how families could participate would be provided, both in written form and in family orientation meetings.

4. Background information would be requested from the family.

5. Education about mental illness, support groups, and family skills training for dealing with a relative who has a mental illness would be provided for families; alternatively, referrals would be offered as to where such education and support could be found.

6. A forum would be established whereby periodic exchanges between family members and treatment staff would occur in order to:

   • inform the family of the current focus of treatment and what the family could do to support it
   • share concerns about the patient's progress
   • update one another on discharge plans

7. Whenever treatment planning conferences were held, consideration would be given to inviting family members or soliciting input from the family. Significant results of such conferences would be conveyed to families when no family member attended.

8. Families would routinely be informed of any significant changes in the status of a client in the program.

This process could easily be instituted without disclosing the details of any personal information that patients divulge in individual or group sessions. Families usually do not want that type of information, nor do they need to have it. They need and want only to have a general idea of what type of treatment or services their relative is receiving, what they can do to support them, and when their relative is likely to be discharged. Similarly, it is to the advantage of the program staff to know what kind of interactions are occurring between consumers and their families. Obtaining an authorization for release of information will take care of issues of confidentiality between the facility and families.

Our mental-health system is currently grossly lacking in resources and funds, but I am convinced that it can be improved by families and providers joining forces and resources. By following the guidelines offered in this chapter and in the Quick Reference Guides, you will have a better chance of getting the best services for your relative that are currently available in this country. As I have repeatedly emphasized, you must know what you can realistically expect and how to deal with the people and facilities that exist.

9

Dealing with
Practical Matters
Housing, Jobs, Money, and Stigma

THE CONCERNS AND NEEDS that face people with mental illness, their friends, and family are more than enough for anyone to deal with. They are not, unfortunately, the end of the problems that demand your attention. There remain issues related to external and practical matters such as what to say to friends, relatives, neighbors, and coworkers about your relative's illness and the problems it raises in your life. Other issues involve providing the assistance your relative may need in dealing with financial matters and looking for suitable housing or work. In each of these arenas you will frequently encounter the ignorance and prejudice that surround mental illness and create the stigma. This chapter offers suggestions for dealing with these problems.

TALKING TO OUTSIDERS

Most stereotypes and prejudice about mental illness are based on a lack of accurate information or firsthand experience. Consequently, the best way to respond to outsiders you en-

FIGHTING STIGMA AND
FOSTERING ACCEPTANCE

Prejudice and stigma are based on ignorance and myths. The best antidote is education or firsthand experience. You are in an ideal position to provide people with some basic information to lessen fears, dispel misconceptions, and open their hearts to those struggling with mental illness. When speaking with people about mental illness, keep the following in mind:

- Mental illnesses have a strong biological component.
- Mental illnesses affect thinking, behavior, feeling, and judgment.
- People's functioning fluctuates greatly.
- Mental illnesses are not contagious or dangerous.
- Mental illnesses are extremely widespread. Over six million Americans suffer from them, and occupy more hospital beds than patients with cancer, diabetes, arthritis, and heart disease combined.
- Medical science is quite ignorant about mental illnesses. There is no known cause, cure, or prevention.
- Treatments can reduce symptoms, at times, for some people, just as with cancer or diabetes.
- Mental illnesses are extremely severe, and often prone to relapse.
- Mental illnesses put enormous emotional and financial strain on families and the country.

- There is woefully little money available for research, services, and treatment facilities.

Remember that you can explain in varying degrees of detail your situation and that of your relative; you need not explain to everyone every aspect of your problem.

You need and deserve compassion and support. Your acceptance of the illness can inspire friends and relatives to do the same. Fight prejudice and stigma and improve conditions for people with mental illness by any of the following modes of action:

- Continue to educate yourself and others.
- Maintain and convey as accepting and compassionate an attitude as possible.
- Participate in national, state, and local chapters of NAMI.
- Actively respond to prejudicial or incorrect information in the media or among friends and relatives.
- Write letters to legislators supporting increased funding, improved health-care conditions, and so forth.
- Volunteer to work with agencies serving people who have mental illnesses or with support groups for families and friends.
- Offer support to families struggling with similar situations.
- Mobilize any special talents or resources you have (writing, filmmaking, artwork) to foster education about and compassion for people with mental illnesses.

counter is by speaking out knowledgeably. The Quick Reference Guide, Fighting Stigma and Fostering Acceptance, summarizes the information that can help you correct most of the misperceptions you will encounter in the general public.

It is unfortunate that in addition to everything else with which you have to contend, you also have to educate people about mental illness. On the one hand, you already have so much stress in your life that you have little energy left over for this task. On the other hand, your firsthand experience puts you in the position of being able to speak with authority and compassion. Those who care about you will likely pay attention to what you say because they are concerned about the needs of your family.

You may find it useful to prepare several ways of describing your situation. You can then choose the way that best suits your mood and the situation. When you are with close friends or relatives, you might give detailed explanations of what has happened to your ill relative and the impact it has had on you and the rest of your family. You may want to share the diagnosis, prognosis, and any information you have learned about mental illnesses, as well as the confusion, heartache, and sadness that you have experienced.

With people you do not know very well, or with neighbors, you may want to give a very abridged version. They may need to know only that your son is suffering from a biological illness that sometimes affects the way he behaves. You can assure them that he is not dangerous and tell them that they ought to just say hello if they see him outside, even if he appears to be talking to himself.

Think also about such situations as what to tell coworkers who may answer the phone when your ill relative calls. You need not say more than that he is ill, in crisis at times, and that you would like to talk to him whenever he calls. When you run into former friends of yours or of your ill relative, remember that you can give as much or as little information as you like. You can say your relative has been having a hard time but you don't feel like talking about the situation. Or you can go into detail, discussing the diagnosis and a summary of his or her history. The only rule is to do whatever works best for you.

People will usually follow your lead regarding how much to discuss the situation. Do not expect your friends to ask how your ill son is doing if you never bring up the subject yourself. It is wise to assume that most people who care about you want to be sensitive to you and to your family, but it is also wise to assume that most people do not have a clue as to how to do so. People with a relative who has a mental illness often feel hurt by friends who feel awkward about the situation and, with the best of intentions, say or do the wrong thing.

Educating your friends, colleagues, and relatives puts yet another burden on you, but this is one I strongly encourage you to embrace, at least for a few important people in your life. Otherwise you will find yourself in the all-too-common position of feeling further isolated and resentful of friends and relatives. Deciding you cannot talk to anyone about one of the most significant parts of your life is bound to take its toll. Most of your friends and relatives need to hear no more than a few of the basic facts outlined in the preceding Quick Reference Guide. If they want to learn more, give them this book or some of the information listed in the Resource Directory.

Telling people how they can be supportive of you is also important. You need to spell out whether you want your friends and relatives to ask you about the situation. If it is not helpful to you for people to offer advice, you must tell them so. Let them know whether their efforts to cheer you up feel good.

You may want to tell your friends and relatives that, in many of the following ways, dealing with a mental illness is like dealing with diabetes or cancer.

- The symptoms can be intermittent.
- No one is sure exactly what causes the illnesses.
- There are a number of different kinds of cancer, diabetes, affective disorders, and schizophrenia.
- Some cases are much more severe than others.
- There is a significant hereditary factor.
- There are no known cures.
- There are treatments that help some people.
- The side effects of treatments can be extremely unpleasant.
- The illnesses are very serious and often have a devastating impact on the lives of not only the people who are ill but also those close to them.
- People with a mental illness and those close to them consequently need a great deal of support and understanding.

Today most people are familiar with cancer and diabetes, and it is now socially acceptable to talk about those illnesses. Most people have a better sense of how to be supportive of friends and relatives of cancer patients and people with diabetes. Thus, by comparing mental illness with cancer or diabetes, you may give people a better idea of what you are going through and how they can be supportive of you.

Another way for you to help fight the ignorance, stigma, and prejudice that surround mental illness is through participation in NAMI. Many local chapters as well as the state and national groups are very involved in a campaign to eradicate the stigma associated with mental illness. Some set up media watches to respond to television, radio, magazine, and newspaper stories that give either inaccurate or biased information about mental illnesses. The alliance is also involved in educating both the public and professionals about mental illness. Its legislative committees are involved in both developing and lobbying for local and national legislation that affects people with mental illness and their families. If you think you would find this kind of involvement satisfying, NAMI could be a most effective outlet for your energy.

It is also important to keep in mind the limitations on how much you can change relatives, friends, and the general public. Often family members who become active in fighting for the rights of people with mental illness want everyone in their family to do the same. As I discussed in earlier chapters, it is essential that each family member respect the ways in which other family members are currently dealing with the situation. Never forget that no matter how much a relative tries to distance himself or herself from a relative with a mental illness, he or she cannot escape the impact entirely. Everyone has to go through his or her own journey of coming to terms with an ill relative. The path and pace will differ significantly from one person to another.

APPLYING FOR JOBS AND HOUSING

There is federal legislation designed to protect various groups, including people with disabilities, from discrimination in areas including employment and housing. Title VIII of the Civil Rights Act of 1968 (Fair Housing Act) and the 1990 Americans with Disabilities Act (ADA) are two that families should know about. Most governmental regulations define an individual with a disability as a person who has a physical or mental impairment that substantially limits one or more major life activities, such as walking, talking, hearing, seeing, learning, performing manual tasks, caring for oneself, thinking, concentrating, and interacting with others.

The ADA acknowledges that the continuing existence of unfair discrimination and prejudice denies people with disabilities the opportunity to compete on an equal basis and costs the country billions of dollars in expenses resulting from dependency and non-productivity. The stated purpose of the ADA is to prohibit discrimination on the basis of disability, to assure equality of opportunity, full participation, independent living, and economic self-sufficiency for disabled individuals, and to provide clear, strong, consistent, enforceable standards by which discrimination can be determined.

The part most relevant to people with psychiatric disabilities, Title I of the ADA, applies to private employers with fifteen or more employees, state and local governments, services funded by the government, employment agencies, and labor unions. It prohibits them from discriminating against *qualified individuals* with disabilities in job application procedures, hiring, firing, advancement, compensation, job training, and other terms and privileges of employment. The ADA requires that employers provide *reasonable accommodation* to the known physical or mental limitations of a qualified individual with a disability, unless to do so would impose an *undue hardship* on the employer's business.

A *qualified employee* or applicant with a disability is one who, with or without reasonable accommodation, can perform the essential functions of the job. Some *reasonable accommodations* that apply to people with psychiatric disabilities are job restructuring, part-time or modified work schedules, reassignment to a vacant position, or appropriate adjustment or modifications of examinations, training materials, or policies. Universities and colleges often have an office for disabled students. There assistance can be obtained with getting needed reasonable accommodations made so students can complete courses. *Undue hardship* is defined as an action requiring significant difficulty or expense, considering factors such as an employer's size, financial resources, and the nature of its operation. An employer is not required to lower quality or production standards to make an accommodation.

Employers may not ask job applicants about the existence, nature, or severity of a disability. Applicants may be asked about their ability to perform specific job functions. Employees and applicants currently engaging in the illegal use of drugs are not covered by the ADA.

The Fair Housing Act covers most housing though may exempt some, such as small, owner-occupied buildings. It prohibits discrimination, such as refusing to rent or sell housing, making housing unavailable, setting different terms or privileges for sale or rental of a dwelling, falsely denying that housing is available for sale or rental, and denying access to or membership in services related to the sale or rental of housing.

If discrimination occurs in housing or employment, complaints can be filed by calling the Department of Housing and Urban Development (HUD) at 1-800-669-9777 or the Equal Employment Opportunity Commission at 1-800-669-4000 to find a local office.

If we had all the funding necessary for services for people with a mental illness, families would not have to get involved in the process of helping a relative with a mental illness find a job or a place to live. Instead, such practical matters would be handled by a case manager, social worker, or vocational counselor. In some areas such resources are available, but in most the family winds up doing the job. The Quick Reference Guide, Filling Out Job and Housing Applications, outlines the essentials for most such situations.

It is a good idea to encourage the ill person to be as actively involved in the application process as he or she can.

Think of yourself as a coach rather than as the one looking for a job or apartment. It is also wise for you to assume that the ill person will be anxious about or fearful of the process. He or she will likely need a lot of reassurance or encouragement. For moral support, you may want to drive the person to and from interviews. Dress rehearsals are extremely useful. Pretend that you are the landlord or employer. Have the person go through the entire process, from initial contact to acceptance or rejection. Praise all efforts, even if the outcome is disappointing. Otherwise you run the risk that your relative will give up altogether.

FINANCIAL MATTERS

Dealing with money can be an enormous problem for people with mental illness. They may have difficulty obtaining money to which they are entitled, and they may be unable to manage money once they get it.

There are some public monies available to help with living expenses and treatment for people with a mental illness, such as Supplemental Security Income (SSI), Social Security Disability Insurance (SSDI), General Assistance (GA), and Medicaid. Unfortunately, the government does not make this money easily accessible and does not take into account the nature of mental illnesses. The fact that thinking, judgment, and the ability to be organized are impaired by mental illnesses makes it impossible for some people who are eligible for support to obtain it. To be eligible for SSI, for instance, a person with a mental illness has to swear, under penalty of perjury, that he or she is unable to work and will continue to be unable to work for twelve months due to a mental disorder. This is difficult for those people who suffer from mental illness yet do not believe they have a mental illness. Others

FILLING OUT JOB AND HOUSING APPLICATIONS

Responding to questions on an application can be a very sensitive, tricky task for people who have been clients in the mental-health system, have gaps in employment history, have been hospitalized, or are on medication. Much depends on the situation and what each individual is comfortable with.

Legally, an employer can ask about a disability only to the extent that it might impede job functions. Therefore, one need elaborate on a disability only if it does impede job performance. Résumés can be written without giving specific dates by using phrases like "One year's experience as a dishwasher."

Lying about length of time worked, positions held, and so forth is not advisable because:

1. Lies can be grounds for immediate termination if they are discovered.
2. Lies often cause anxiety and confusion, which can lead to trouble, including presenting inconsistent information.

Following are some possible ways to word answers about:

- *hospitalization:* "Yes, I was hospitalized for a medical disorder. I needed time to recuperate."
- *gaps between jobs:* "I was participating in a rehabilitation program"; "I was brushing up on some vocational skills"; "I was in a training program"; "I was taking some courses."

continued on following page

continued from previous page

- *income:* (on rental applications): "I have a guaranteed disability income." If asked for further details, responding that one has a medical disability usually discourages further inquiry.
- *medication:* most medication can be described as a way to help control nerves or anxiety (many antipsychotic medications are classified as major tranquilizers) or to help boost energy (antidepressants).

Employers or landlords who are going to discriminate against people for looking different or for having a mental-health history will usually do so early on in the process. Phone screening can eliminate many face-to-face rejections and wounds caused by discrimination.

It is helpful for people applying for jobs or housing to be coached and to rehearse. What is considered appropriate dress and behavior is not always apparent to people with mental illness. Rather than filling out applications on the spot, it is better for them to be filled out in advance. It is also wise to have duplicates ready in case more than one is required, one gets lost or soiled, or another opportunity arises. Landlords curious as to what someone who receives disability income does during the day are usually satisfied to hear that the person is enrolled in a school or vocational or training program. References need to be considered in advance. Relatives can attest to the person's ability to make regular payment of rent or to the person's level of responsibility if they are familiar with those aspects of the person's life.

are very ashamed of having a mental illness, or are too proud to go on welfare. Still others are too confused to be able to swear to anything or to be sure about what will happen in the next hour, let alone in the next twelve months.

Government bureaucracies can be frustrating and infuriating for even the healthiest college graduate. They often pose insurmountable obstacles for people with mental illness, who generally are not patient or level-headed enough to see their way through the application process. Filling out forms and being interviewed can be stressful, complicated, and confusing. Additionally, applicants must have an address to which checks can be sent. People who have a mental illness and are homeless or transient cannot always provide an address where they can consistently receive mail.

In the best of all worlds social workers or case managers would help disabled people through the governmental red tape. Since this is so often not the case, you may have to contact the local Social Security or social-services office to find out what financial and medical benefits are available in your area and how to apply for them. Then be prepared to help your ill relative through the entire process. It is an extremely rare person suffering with a mental illness who can handle applying for SSI or for admission to the state medical program without help.

The Quick Reference Guide, Options for Financing Living and Treatment Expenses, outlines the types of arrangements and programs available to help pay for the living and treatment expenses of people with mental illness.

In finances, as in other areas described in this book, it is best for ill people to assume as much responsibility for themselves as they can. Since the risks are high when it comes to money, more assistance will probably be required. Without properly managing money, it may be impossible to maintain a decent housing situation, participation in a treatment program, and compliance with medication. Thus, dealing with money may well warrant some assistance if the ill person cannot handle it himself or herself. Difficulty in dealing with finances and the corresponding red tape is among the major factors, along with the lack of funding for adequate services and the lack of affordable housing, that contribute to the high rate of homelessness among people with mental illness.

Many families want their ill relative to have access to public support so that they can keep whatever financial resources the family has in reserve for additional goods and services to increase the ill person's quality of life. While this is a humane goal, it is not always easily accomplished and may require sophisticated financial planning. If your family has some financial resources available, it is crucial that you consult one of the relevant books mentioned in the Resource Directory or see an attorney with expertise in this highly specialized area to find out how best to provide some security for your relative both before and after your death. The laws vary from state to state. Families of people with developmental disabilities have been working on this for decades. They have cleared a path that families of people with mental illness are following. Planning can help you avoid the pain experienced by families who, failing to think ahead, wind up watching enormous sums of money disappear and then find their relative left with nothing.

I have tried to present in this book everything that most people are likely to need to know about mental illness and caring for a relative with a mental illness. Those who are more intimately involved with someone with a major mental illness probably need much more information than any single book can provide, and I encourage them to use the additional resources I have listed.

My heart goes out to those of you who have a loved one with a mental illness. You need an enormous amount of courage and stamina just to contend with the demands of your everyday lives. Please remember that your lives are far more stressful than those of most other people. You therefore need and deserve extra support and assistance to truly thrive.

OPTIONS FOR FINANCING LIVING AND TREATMENT EXPENSES

Living expenses can be financed by one or more of the following:

1. SSI (Supplemental Security Income): for people unable to work for at least twelve months due to a disability, including a mental disorder

2. SSDI (Social Security Disability Insurance): for people who have had previous work experience and cannot currently work

3. Veterans Administration pension (for veterans)

4. savings or trust fund

5. family support

Treatment can be financed by one or more of the following:

1. state or federal medical programs, such as Medicare (for those over 65) and Medicaid

2. county medical programs (for those ineligible for state programs)

continued on following page

continued from previous page

3. private medical insurance (though companies often limit benefits for mental illnesses)
4. Veterans Administration benefits (for veterans)
5. state-funded mental-health programs
6. private agencies or agencies under county contracts
7. private funds

How money, decisions about living, and treatment are made depends, in part, on:

1. who is designated as the payee
2. whether there is a conservator or legal guardian who has the authority to control a person's money or mandate treatment

Some ways to handle finances:

1. Parents, spouse (or some other responsible authority) can handle all monies. This minimizes risks, but maximizes dependence and interpersonal problems.
2. A relative or payee can pay some essential bills (like rent) and give the ill person an allowance.
3. The ill person can handle all monies. This arrangement maximizes both independence and risks.

It is advisable to move from option 1 to option 3 in very small steps as the ill person demonstrates an ability to handle increasing financial responsibility.

You can arrange for the future security of your relative by:

1. leaving money to others who will provide for your relative's needs
2. having a relative or friend control a trust fund
3. having a nonprofit organization control a trust fund. NAMI has established a Guardian and Trusts Network. This group has information about estate planning and organizations that provide caregiving services when the family is no longer around. To find out if such an organization has been set up in your state, contact the Network through NAMI, 2107 Wilson Blvd., Suite 300, Arlington, Virginia, 22201-3042 (703) 524-7600
4. setting up a bank trust
5. leaving housing to the person

Please do not allow pride or shame to prevent you from finding people with whom and places where you can talk about the myriad problems that life with someone who has a mental illness presents.

Also, please do not fault yourself for not knowing more about mental illness than you do. Until fairly recently, this information has been unavailable. If you feel bad or angry about your lack of knowledge, try not to turn those feelings against you or those close to you. Instead, use your energy to educate someone else in need or to fight for more funding for research and services for people with mental illness and their families. There is much work to be done, and you have already suffered more than you deserve.

We can improve the lives of people with mental illness and their families only when all of us who care band together, raise our voices, and demand that a greater priority be given to funding research and services for those suffering from these most mysterious, cruel, and disabling illnesses.

10

Recovery from Mental Illness and Understanding and Responding to Dual Disorders

RECOVERY FROM MENTAL ILLNESS

Consumers have discussed and written extensively about ways in which their friends, family, and providers of services can best support them in living as full and meaningful lives as possible. Doing this often entails a change in attitudes. Rather than regarding people as mental patients devastated by a disease, we must see them as competent human beings struggling to live productive lives and experiencing many different kinds of needs. As with everyone, attention must be paid not only to their physical health needs but also to their spiritual, social, cultural, and psychological well-being. Consumers advocate a more holistic view of recovery from mental illness, and they find it most helpful when those around them understand and support a recovery model.

When used in relation to mental illness the term "recovery" has a different meaning from that used by people recovering from substance abuse. People recovering from both can find ways to take advantage of both definitions. Consumers of mental-health services talk about the following five sets of experiences from which they need to recover. 1) The symptoms of the illness. 2) Traumas occurring before or during the onset of symptoms. Sometimes these traumas are restimulated when people are restrained, arrested, or mistreated during the course of getting care. 3) The problematic effects of getting no treatment, inadequate treatment, or the wrong type of treatment. 4) The stigma and discrimination associated with mental illness. 5) Ineffective patterns of behaviors developed to cope with the other four.

The process of recovering from mental illness has both internal and external components. One must regain pride, self-esteem, and an identity as a unique, worthwhile, competent person with potential for growth. Internal changes in perspective are enhanced by supportive interactions with others, be they fellow consumers, caring providers, loving family, or friends. The essential elements are being there, seeing the whole person, and reflecting that back to them in a positive, compassionate, and hopeful way. It makes an enormous difference to people suffering—physically, spiritually, and emotionally—to know that there is someone who believes in them even through their darkest hours when they do not believe in themselves, and to know that someone will be there with them for the long haul, through good times and bad.

For many people spirituality, feeling connected to something bigger than themselves and their illness, is an essential part of their recovery. It is not important what kind of spiritual practice or religious affiliation a person has as long as they are accepted for who they are. Being part of almost any supportive faith community can offer enormous comfort and help an individual maintain a more positive perspective.

The external component of recovery includes involvement with work or other meaningful activities, friends, housing, and material goods that may have been lost in the course of the illness. Consumers believe that finding a meaningful niche in life and a way to be part of the larger community is essential to recovery. There are also functions, including life skills, such as cooking, cleaning, and keeping a checking account, communication skills, and the capacity to sleep well, that need to be recovered.

Consumers feel extremely passionate about recovery from mental illness. This change in attitude and approach brings with it a beginning or returning to a life filled with pride, hopes, and dreams for the future. It provides opportunities to learn and grow from the pain and suffering endured. It supports people in rediscovering who they are and all they can be despite their symptoms and possible limitations. It counteracts the stigma and negativism that society has inflicted upon individuals with psychiatric disorders.

Consumers have found several ways to rebuild and find meaning in their lives. Some discover it through creative arts, others through sharing their experience and recovery with people struggling with a similar illness. Still others find purpose through educational pursuits, volunteer projects, or paid work. What is important is determining a way to be productive, competent, or making a contribution to society. It is useful for family and caregivers to help people find their unique areas of strength and methods of expression.

Among the most crucial aspects of the consumer movement are self-responsibility, empowerment, and self-determination. People who do best living with a mental illness need to do more than merely accept that they have an illness or that something is wrong with them. They need to find ways to take charge of their lives and treatment. Family and caregivers can be most helpful by believing in people, being hopeful, and encouraging them to take responsibility for their lives. One way to do this is to encourage consumers to contact other consumers and consumer groups. Local groups can be found through the National Mental Health Consumers' Self-Help Clearinghouse at *www.mhselfhelp.org*, a local NAMI group, or the National Mental Health Association.

Recovery is an extremely personal process. It is a journey that each person travels in his or her own way and time frame. It will be very subtle or gradual for some and more sudden or dramatic for others. This journey is not linear. It will inevitably take many twists, turns, and forward and backward movement. There may be times, especially in the beginning, when the person feels confused, discouraged, isolated, ineffective, and hopeless. It is very important to have others along the way who believe in the person, have hope for his or her future, and help him or her remember, and attain some of his or her dreams and goals.

While no one may be able to prevent the symptoms from recurring or cure the illness, people can learn to take charge of their lives. When people begin to take responsibility for developing coping skills and learning ways to manage their illness, they have taken a significant step forward. It is when focusing on what they can do to improve their quality of life that things often begin to get better.

Caregivers are most helpful when they collaborate with people in meeting goals consumers set for themselves. While doing this, consumers must consistently be treated with humanity and respect for the struggles in which they engage. Caregivers can also assist by offering education about mental illness, substance abuse, recovery, services available, medication, other forms of treatment, and the pros and cons of each. This will aid consumers in making informed decisions.

There is a delicate balance to be achieved. We want to move away from the view of people as helpless victims of an illness. We want to encourage people to assume responsibility for their lives and decisions that affect them. We do not, however, want to give the message that everyone is always able to make the best choices for themselves with no outside assistance.

Many discussions have taken place about whether or not people who have an illness that impairs their cognitive functioning are always able to make the best decisions for themselves. On the one hand, most adults feel they have the right to make choices for themselves and to experience the consequences. Consumers advocate for the "dignity of risk and right to fail." On the other hand, society and families often feel they should protect and make decisions for those unable to take care of themselves. There is no simple answer, and future discussion will no doubt continue to bring changes in laws and how they are implemented, and to the delivery of services. Those in the consumer movement, who call for all consumers to have complete control over all decisions affecting them, tend to be more consistently high-functioning people. The families who most ardently disagree usually have relatives who are more consistently lower-functioning, unable to take care of themselves, and unable to make decisions that most people would deem beneficial ones that allow them to have the best possible quality of life. For example, they may refuse all treatment and, consequently, live very marginal lives on the streets.

It seems there is not one solution that applies to all people in all situations. The crucial factors to consider are how well people are able to function, how severe their symptoms are, how much insight they have into their illness, their safety, and the quality and accessibility of treatment and services. A person living independently who understands his illness and symptoms and decides to stop taking medication for a few days is very different from one who does not understand he is ill, has severe symptoms that do not allow him to take care of himself, and refuses all forms of treatment.

The mental-health service system needs to be expanded

and revamped to better meet consumers' needs. One way consumers, family, and caregivers can help is by advocating for more government funding for services and research. NAMI is a good resource regarding legislation currently being considered and developed. While systems have improved, they have a long way to go. More ways to include consumers in designing the system and delivering services need to be developed. Some counties are beginning to hire consumers as peer counselors and consultants to help with this. Having consumers serve as mentors and role models for those just beginning to learn how to manage their own recovery is also essential.

Systems should revolve around stated consumer needs for housing, meaningful employment, and other support services rather than merely continuing to fund pre-existing programs. Consumers appreciate family members and providers who assume a role more as a coach, guide, or teacher instead of as an all-knowing, all-powerful, paternalistic figure, as doctors have previously taken on in "medical model" systems. It is also important that providers collaborate with family, friends, and all who are integral to the consumer's support system. To summarize the importance of their involvement, consumers and families developed the slogan, "Nothing about us, without us."

Consumers also want providers to be sensitive to the different cultures from which they and their families come.

CULTURAL SENSITIVITY

Many countries have a variety of diverse communities or subcultures coexisting within them. In the United States for example, there are many Asian-Americans, African-Americans, Hispanics, Native Americans, and others. Each of these subcultures has somewhat different understandings of mental illness, substance abuse, caretaking responsibility, and spirituality. In addition, they have different problem-solving styles and relationships to authority. There are efforts being made on the part of service providers to be more culturally sensitive. They do not, however, always know how best to do this, as they are not always familiar with the culture from which a person comes. It is advisable for families not born in this country to inform providers of how long you have been here and the circumstances of your immigration.

The degree of independence or interdependence within a family varies greatly in different cultures. The value placed on individuality and independence in mainstream American culture goes far beyond that of most other countries in the world and subcultures within the U.S. Providers may need to be reminded that in other cultures the level of family involvement is normally quite extensive. In many cultures, family is the most important core value and foundation in life. Family is often defined more broadly than in the U.S., where the nuclear family is the primary, sometimes exclusive, unit involved with the caretaking of ill relatives. In other cultures, there are larger extended families that may include people who are not blood relatives.

In many Asian and Hispanic cultures it is natural for unmarried adults to live with their parents and families of origin and to be taken care of in ways that are less common in the United States. In urban settings, recommendations are often made that consumers live outside the family to get the best care. This may produce great discomfort in many families, being perceived as an act of disloyalty or an insinuation of inadequacy on the part of a family. It also may be less appropriate when there is no one in the alternative placement who speaks the language or is familiar with the food and culture of the consumer.

Providers should make efforts to understand how problems are typically solved in different cultures. It should be ascertained if problems are solved democratically, by an individual matriarch, patriarch, or other decision maker, by a group of "elders," or in another manner. Care providers must learn the hierarchy in each family and make special efforts to include the important person or persons in all the major decisions regarding the consumer. Without such involvement, any plan developed may be ineffective.

There are two major taboos with which many families have to contend. One is to accept that serious mental illness and substance abuse are occurring in the family. Neither may be understood as an illness that can be treated. For many cultures there is an enormous amount of disgrace and shame associated with having either psychiatric symptoms or substance-abuse problems. The other taboo is the notion of turning outside the family for help. Doing so may be seen as weak, unacceptable, or, at best, a last resort.

Mental illness and substance abuse are understood by some cultures as resulting from possession by evil spirits, the devil, or as the will of God. For Hispanics, symptoms of mental illness may be considered a "nervous problem." They may be seen as character weaknesses, which should be kept hidden or dealt with only within the family.

Many Asian-Americans tend to understand mental illness or substance abuse as being caused by external factors, such as stress or the bad influence of others. They may experience a family member's inability to function as extremely shameful, and fear losing face. The family's reaction to a member who is exhibiting symptoms may be to isolate or scold them. They might send the person back to the country of origin or disown them entirely. It takes time, respect, and sensitivity to help such a family overcome these barriers and accept some of what Western treatments have to offer.

If willing to seek help outside the family, Asian families

might first go to an herbalist or someone with a holistic approach. Hispanic families might go to a "curandero" to provide healing. African-Americans might turn to their clergy. Any of these can be included in a care plan with the consumer and Western service providers.

Many African-Americans and people from other minority cultures have developed an understandable mistrust in "the system." This is based on insensitive or racist interactions they have had in the past. Providers must strive not to be offended or pushed away by families that need to test them or initially challenge them. It may be a way for them to determine if previous bad experiences are going to be repeated. Not everyone will immediately be a passive, submissive, or grateful recipient of a provider's time. It would be helpful for families to let a new provider know if they have had bad previous experiences with providers.

Asian families and consumers may need to educate providers about what is comfortable in terms of eye contact and personal space. Westerners tend to stand closer and make more eye contact than is customary in most Asian cultures. This may be experienced as disrespectful or rude.

Families must understand that not all providers take into account the importance of religion and spirituality in many cultures. Providers must remember that spirituality is a source of great strength, comfort, and healing. It would be wise for providers to learn about the place religion plays in the culture of people with whom they work. Many families and individuals in need have accessed services only when providers and families partnered with local church leaders or other important members of the community.

In some urban areas there are mental-health centers that specialize in serving people from particular cultures. They have staff that speak the primary language of the consumers and understand the cultures from which they come. This is the ideal. When this is not the case, families and consumers may be put off by a system that appears, in its ignorance, to be insensitive to their basic values. Families are encouraged to try not to completely reject such service providers. While they may have much to learn about your particular culture, they may also have something to offer the consumer and the family. Providers have to selectively modify services and recommendations so that they are more compatible with the culture from which the family and consumer come.

When providers and families are of different cultural backgrounds, each must make an effort to understand the values and beliefs of the other. Each must be respectful and open to learning from the other. It is when cultural differences are acknowledged that ways to blend Western treatments with other frameworks can be found. Families are an invaluable source of strength and support for individuals with serious problems. They must figure out how to provide what they can while also utilizing available services. While it takes additional time for family members and providers to get to know one another and develop trust, it is time well spent as it almost inevitably insures the best possible results for the consumer. Providers, family, and friends need to partner with consumers to assist them in achieving their own realistic, positive goals.

WRAP

Mary Ellen Copeland developed a tool that is increasingly being used by consumers. It has been particularly helpful in providing a system consumers can use to monitor their own recovery and lives. It is called a Wellness Recovery Action Plan, or WRAP for short. Ms. Copeland has written a WRAP booklet describing how to use the plan for dealing with physical and emotional symptoms, and another specifically for people with dual disorders. While a WRAP must be written by the person who will use it, it does emphasize the importance of supporters. Therefore, it is wise for caregivers and family members of people who might use WRAP to become familiar with it.

There are a number of basic values upon which the WRAP is based. The plan has no predetermined definition for wellness, recognizing the importance of each person defining this for himself or herself. It can be used alongside any other forms of treatment or services. It is not meant to replace other forms of treatment. It assumes every person is unique, special, and has no limits to their recovery. It is designed as a way to empower people to actively participate in improving their lives and the care they receive. It is a beautiful manifestation of the recovery and consumer empowerment movement, as it begins with and maintains a strong focus on a person's strengths while also setting up ways to handle problems, symptoms, and crises.

There are five basic parts to a WRAP. First the person lists a description of what he or she does and what she or he is like when feeling well, without symptoms. The person develops a wellness toolbox. These tools, such as talking with a friend or relative or exercising, are used to help the person stay well and help relieve symptoms. A daily maintenance plan is developed. This begins with a list of all the positive traits and skills a person has. It also includes all the daily activities a person does when things are going well. It is useful to remind oneself of these when things begin to feel bad. Throughout, the important thing is that the person writing the plan decides what tools are useful, and when and how much to use them.

The second section consists of a list of triggers. These may be external events, experiences, or feelings that have historically upset the person and precipitated symptoms or substance abuse. These might include things such as having an argument with a friend or relative, developing a physical illness, or having a birthday. This part also presents a trigger plan. This is a list of things the person can do when triggers occur, such as writing in a journal or going to a twelve-step meeting.

In section three, the person lists the early warning signs of their illness. These tend to be internal and unrelated to external events. They may occur in spite of all efforts to reduce stress. They include all subtle and not-so-subtle changes that indicate the need for further action. Examples are withdrawing from people, avoiding things on the daily maintenance list, feeling more irritable, and changes in eating or sleeping habits. Action plans are detailed in this section as well. They might include taking extra medication or doing things on the daily maintenance plan even if one does not feel like it. This part is designed to remind the person of ways to prevent their condition from getting worse.

The next section is a list of symptoms, unique to each individual, that indicates things are getting pretty bad. This is a time when immediate action is called for to prevent a full-blown crisis. The list usually includes some symptoms or problematic behaviors, such as substance abuse or discontinuing the use of medications that are known to be effective. Again, the person writes a list of actions that should be taken to avoid a crisis. Usually this involves contacting someone the person trusts to help him or her get back on track.

In the final section, a crisis plan is written. This needs to be done when a person is well. It is a way for the person to inform her support system of her wishes in the event of a crisis in which she is (temporarily) unable to take responsibility for her own care. It begins with a description of what she is like when well. Then there is a list of symptoms which indicate the need for others to take over. This is often the most difficult part for a person to write. Finally, the person records who she wants contacted, where she prefers to receive treatment, and what kind of involvement she wants from others. The person also makes a list of indicators that she no longer needs this level of help. For example, being able to sleep through the night, being able to take care of personal hygiene, or being able to carry on a good conversation might be on the list. As with each part of the plan, it will be very individual. No two will be alike.

While all caregivers should support and encourage a person who writes a WRAP, it is equally important that family members not pressure a person to use such a tool specifically designed to help one take charge of one's own life. WRAP has many similarities to the type of relapse-prevention planning discussed on page 241 and the kind that has long been used in substance-abuse programs. It is a good example of how care for both major psychiatric disorders and substance-use disorders can be handled in a consistent manner. For more information on WRAP, see Mary Ellen Copeland's website: *www.mentalhealthrecovery.com,* or phone (802) 254-2092.

SUBSTANCE ABUSE DEFINED

How does a family know whether or not their loved one has a substance-abuse problem? Many experts believe that for someone who is also recovering from a serious psychiatric disability, any use of street drugs, alcohol, or prescription medication other than as prescribed, constitutes abuse. This is because it is likely to trigger or increase psychiatric symptoms. Determining whether someone with a major psychiatric disorder also has a serious substance-use problem is complicated by many factors, particularly the following two. Firstly, everyone who abuses substances tends to deny, minimize, and hide the fact that they do so. Secondly, all the primary symptoms of major psychiatric disorders, psychosis, depression, mania, and anxiety, can occur as a result of using drugs and/or alcohol and from stopping such use. There are a small percentage of people with serious mental illness who are able to use alcohol socially or occasionally with no adverse effects. For most people, however, the risks involved far outweigh the benefits.

It is difficult to assess whether someone who abuses substances also has a co-occurring psychiatric disorder. For long-term drug and alcohol users, the only way to determine if they have a separate diagnosable mental illness is to observe them after being clean and sober for at least a year. Only if symptoms persist afterward can an accurate diagnosis be made. Because many long-term addicts are not willing or able to remain clean and sober for even six months, they and their loved ones may never be able to obtain an accurate psychiatric diagnosis. Nonetheless, people should be treated for psychiatric symptoms when they occur.

Making the assessment, as to whether a person has both a substance-use problem and a separate serious mental illness, is best done by a professional well trained and experienced in both areas. Many programs and professionals claiming to work with people with a dual diagnosis primarily see substance abusers with personality disorders or other psychiatric disorders. They are less familiar with people with schizophrenia, schizoaffective disorder, and bipolar disorder. Similarly, many mental-health program staff do not know how to do a thorough substance-abuse assessment or how to treat a serious substance-use disorder.

It is unrealistic for most families to be able to make such a determination. It is useful, however, for families and caregivers to have some familiarity with substance abuse. The intent of this chapter is to provide families and caregivers with basic information about substance abuse and recovery.

The world of substance abuse and recovery has developed a culture and language of its own. It is useful for family and caregivers to become familiar with this. Therefore, throughout this discussion, some of the more commonly used concepts and vocabulary will be presented. When the term "drugs and alcohol" is used, what is being referred to is all street drugs; all forms of alcohol, including beer and wine; prescription medication when taken other than as prescribed or when abused in other ways; and over-the-counter medication when taken in ways, combinations, or doses other than what is recommended. People with substance-use disorders will sometimes abuse anything to which they have access, including substances that others have no idea can be used to get "high." For example, many people are surprised that some herbal remedies, glue, paint, or chemicals used for cleaning are abused in this way. People will also use such things as cough syrup, mouthwash, and cold tablets to get "high." Even experienced substance-use counselors are astonished by the ever-changing chemicals that people discover can be used to alter their mind or mood.

People who abuse prescription medication become very adept at getting doctors to prescribe what they want. They go to different doctors and dentists, without disclosing their full history, and take medicine beyond prescribed doses. For some addicts, prescription medications, often painkillers or antianxiety medications, are their "drugs of choice." Most addicts prefer one or two types of drugs but will use whatever is most readily available or accessible to them.

Exactly what is substance abuse? The simplest definition was offered in chapter five. This defines abuse as occurring when a person continues to use or drink despite negative consequences. A more extensive description is: **A lifelong, progressive, family disease of denial with a tendency toward relapse.** This encompasses six of the most important things to understand about addiction.

1. For most addicts and alcoholics, including those with many years of recovery and sobriety, addiction is something they need to be vigilant about throughout their lives as the possibility of recurrence is high.

2. Being a progressive disease signifies that it gets worse over time. People's tolerance increases. This means that they need to drink or use increasing amounts to get the same effect. This is true even if one stops using or drinking. If one resumes use, things will not start over from the beginning, but pick up just where they left off. For example, Tom began drinking only a beer or two a night in college. By the time he was twenty-five, he was drinking two six packs a night. By age thirty, he was drinking two six packs and half a pint of vodka a night. He then went into recovery and stopped drinking for ten years. Shortly after he resumed drinking, he again needed to drink two six packs and half a pint of vodka to get the effect he was looking for.

3. It is a disease that inevitably affects all family members and loved ones close to the person. This does not mean that the family is responsible for a person's drug abuse or alcoholism. It does mean that family members need to learn about abuse and how their actions can make things better or worse. There is a hereditary factor that makes people more likely to become addicts if there is a family history of addiction.

4. Being a disease means that there are physiological

changes that occur in the brains of addicts. When addicts use or drink, their ability to stop is physiologically impaired. The brain compels them to continue using, even in place of eating or other necessary activities. The rational part of the mind may see the problems and consequences inherent in continuing to use. However, another more compelling part of the brain craves the substance despite the negative consequences.

5. Denial of the existence or extent of one's dependence or addiction is an inherent part of the disease. The general rule of thumb is to take what an addict tells you about how much they are using and multiply it by five to get a more accurate idea of the truth. A striking and well-known phenomenon among addicts is that, despite repeated negative outcomes, they continue to expect different results each time they use. They continue to maintain, for instance, that this time they will be able to handle their use without anything bad happening to them or to someone close to them.

6. Addiction is said to be a very patient disease. It waits for opportunities to again rear its ugly head. It frequently recurs in people who have been drinking or using extensively for a long time. People rarely stop suddenly and permanently. Families need to understand that, as with mental illness, relapses with substance use are often a part of the recovery process. People can grow and learn from relapses if they are working a program of recovery.

It is the effect of the substance use on the person and the person's life that determines if someone has a serious problem. It is not the quantity consumed, or the duration of use.

The following are some of the many common misconceptions about abuse:

- Waiting until evening to start using means it is not a serious problem.
- Drinking only beer or wine means a person is not an alcoholic.
- Continuing to work and function means a person is not an alcoholic.

People who abuse substances soon lose the ability to control how much they drink or use. They cannot stop after having just one drink even if they intend to. A person's ability to stop after one drink or to limit use of a drug is one part of assessing a substance-use problem.

RECOGNIZING SIGNS OF SUBSTANCE ABUSE

How might family or caregivers know if a person is using? Occasional use may at first seem benign and cause no apparent problems. If it continues and increases, problems inevitably do occur. Family members may notice more or less subtle changes in appearance or behavior. The following is a list of indicators that substance abuse may be occurring:

- changes in behavior
- changes in physical appearance or personal hygiene
- changes in friends
- becoming more secretive
- decreased involvement in responsible activities; becoming less reliable
- lying

- sudden money problems
- money or valuables missing from those in contact with the person
- redness in the eyes; dilated or pinpoint pupils
- the presence of drug paraphernalia
- deterioration in family relationships
- increase in psychiatric symptoms

CENTRAL FOCUS

In order to have compassion for people who abuse substances, it is important to understand what it is like to become addicted physically or psychologically to a substance. One of the most essential aspects of this is to realize that, even without the addict becoming aware of it, the substance or getting "high" on something gradually becomes the most important thing in life. Over time, drinking or using becomes all-consuming and the central focus of time, energy, and money. Life begins to revolve around using and obtaining the money to buy more drugs or alcohol. Most of the time what is going through the minds of addicts has to do with what, when, and where they will next use. They may lose interest in other activities and in spending time with people who do not use or drink. They may engage in behaviors that they and their family could never have imagined, such as trading sex for drugs.

There are stages to addiction that people go through. Gradually dependency increases. As people lose control over their ability to limit their use, many aspects of their lives begin to crumble. In the final stages of drug or alcohol dependence, addicts experience withdrawal symptoms if they do not continue to feed their habit. At this point, they are not using to get high or to feel good but to avoid the terrible physical

238 WHEN SOMEONE YOU LOVE HAS A MENTAL ILLNESS

symptoms they will experience without continued use. This inevitably precipitates deterioration in social, physical, and psychological well-being.

With serious substance abuse comes a host of other behaviors that are considered part of the disease and cause serious problems for family, friends, and caregivers. These behaviors, often referred to as "addict behaviors," arise as a result of people needing to devote so much time and energy to obtaining drugs, or the money to buy them, and a desire to hide the extent of their problems. Addict behaviors include being secretive, deceptive, lying, stealing, and manipulating. Addicts become very adept at these. Often it is difficult for family members to believe that previously more honest, hardworking, or dependable relatives could engage in such activities.

Addicts and alcoholics, when in the middle of their addiction, rarely take responsibility for their actions. Instead, they typically "blame, complain, and explain." They minimize or deny the fact that they use or drink, or that any problems result from it. They explain away problems related to their use and blame others for them. They often feel and portray themselves as innocent, sometimes self-righteous victims.

There is another category of behaviors called "drug-seeking behaviors." This refers to the tendency of addicts and alcoholics to look for a "quick fix" or a way to "get high" when they feel upset, bored, or many other uncomfortable feelings. Their immediate, almost automatic, reaction is to focus attention on doing whatever might be necessary to obtain a mood-altering substance. A particular kind of excitement, often with a clandestine component, accompanies these behaviors and becomes a regular part of a lifestyle to which addicts grow very attached.

Some of these behaviors, people, places, or things associated with using can produce a physiological reaction similar to actually using. For example, people experience a "rush" or "high" just from seeing paraphernalia used when doing drugs. Cravings to use or drink can also be triggered by seeing old drinking buddies or smelling beer on the breath of someone else. These cravings and physical reactions can then set in motion the search for drugs, alcohol, or the money and people to obtain them.

WHY PEOPLE USE

Why would anyone choose to get involved in such a lifestyle? People begin using for a variety of reasons. They do not think about where it will lead them.

Often young people experiment with drugs and alcohol in high school or college. They may do this out of curiosity, for fun, or to make or to keep friends. Peer pressure is very strong, especially for adolescents trying to figure out who they are.

Some people use to reduce stress and to feel better. People may feel bad for a variety of reasons, such as difficulties at work, family problems, financial worries, or medical problems. Others begin using to forget painful experiences, such as repeated sexual, physical, or emotional abuse, or an isolated traumatic event. Many veterans begin using while in military service or after experiencing the horrors of war.

People experiencing psychotic symptoms or disturbances in mood may turn to drugs to reduce these symptoms and the fears that they may have a mental illness. People who are using to find relief from psychiatric symptoms often do not realize the interaction between drugs, alcohol, and mental illness. They may experience some short-term symptom relief, yet have no way of knowing that their use will most likely make their symptoms worse in the long run.

For some people, drugs or alcohol may be the only relief

they can find from their symptoms. This may be due to the fact that available medications do not work for everyone. Other people, because of their symptoms or the complexity of the treatment system, are unable or unwilling to utilize services necessary to obtain medication.

Whatever the initial reasons, once someone begins using drugs or alcohol, there is a different physiological process that occurs in addicts than in others. Non-addicts will reduce or stop using over time, develop other coping strategies, seek other forms of help, or "outgrow" this stage in life once they become more involved in adult responsibilities. Addicts and alcoholics are not able to decrease their use. Instead, their use gradually increases and consumes more of their time, energy, and life.

REACTIONS OF FAMILY AND CAREGIVERS

In chapter six, we discussed the normal range of feeling that families of people with a serious mental illness have. When someone has a dual diagnosis, there are additional feelings and issues that arise. These may occur in reaction to the "addictive behaviors," or to the way people behave when they use. There is often a breach of trust that happens with an addict or alcoholic. When people have been lied to, stolen from, and repeatedly manipulated, it is natural to feel angry, taken advantage of, and mistrustful. Families may need to take a break from the person after such things have occurred. A family may wisely decide to limit the amount of contact they have with a person who is actively using or drinking.

It takes time to rebuild trust. People with a dual diagnosis who become involved in treatment learn this. They begin to understand that it is up to them to prove to their relatives that they are changing and will no longer be involved in addict behaviors. They come to realize that it takes a good deal of time for people who have been hurt by the things they have done to heal and to trust them again.

When the behavior of a relative changes, families may be confused about whether it is due to substance use or mental illness. They are unsure how to respond. This is to be expected. It is a very difficult part of what caregivers need to learn. The differences may be subtle. Only with time and repeated experiences will it become clear which is occurring, and what responses will be most effective. For a person with co-occurring disorders, when one disorder becomes severe the other often will follow.

RELAPSE PREVENTION

Relapse-prevention skills are among the most important that people recovering from dual disorders need to learn. While there is a brief discussion of "minimizing relapses" in chapter four, more detailed information is needed by consumers and caregivers. A similar approach can be used when working on preventing relapses from psychiatric and substance-use disorders. Family and caregivers can be a vital part of the relapse-prevention process. Ideally, people in recovery will share many aspects of the process with the important support people in their lives.

There are three essential parts to relapse prevention: identifying the causes of relapse, recognizing the early warning signs, and developing effective interventions. Each will be discussed in some detail. Throughout, it is important to remember that relapse is a process, not an isolated event. The more knowledgeable people are about warning signs, the more choices they have regarding intervention strategies. People often mistakenly tell themselves or those close to them that they had no idea why they suddenly relapsed. They just happened to walk by a liquor store, or saw an old "using buddy" and decided to indulge. This is probably neither the whole story nor how someone who has learned effective relapse-prevention skills would describe it. Those studying the process of relapse learn to recognize the very early changes in thinking, feeling, and behavior that occur.

The leading causes of relapse for substance abuse are often divided into two categories: internal and external. There are two expressions from the world of recovery from substance abuse, especially twelve-step programs, which summarize these very well. The acronym for one is HALT. The other is "slippery" people, places, and things.

Internal causes of relapse are feelings that seem intolerable such as anger, pain, and sadness. The acronym **HALT** stands for *h*ungry, *a*ngry, *l*onely, and *t*ired. These feelings often contribute to relapse. People in recovery must be mindful of them, as they are frequently red flags signaling the need for interventions.

Three of the most common external causes of relapse are "slippery" people, places, and things. These refer to the people with whom an addict is accustomed to using or drinking, the places that he or she goes when using, and the various paraphernalia associated with drugs and alcohol. For some people just seeing an old "using buddy" or riding a bus in the neighborhood where they used to drink can trigger cravings to use again. To avoid the "slippery slope" of relapse people usually need to learn to avoid going to such places, associating with such people, and having "slippery" things around.

Two other common "triggers" for addicts and alcoholics are unstructured time and money. One of the reasons that most recovery programs are very structured is that many addicts and alcoholics get into trouble when they have unstructured time. They tend to do better when they are busy. When they have nothing to do, feelings of loneliness, emptiness, or boredom arise and the desire to use follows. This can be an even greater problem for people who also have psychiatric symptoms, which, when more acute, may limit things they are able to do. This then puts them at greater risk for using.

Another time many people are at greater risk for relapsing is when they have a sum of money, be it a gift, paycheck, or government benefit check. Addicts develop a strong association between having money and using drugs. Money management is a very important issue for many people with a dual diagnosis. It can determine whether a person is able to live independently. It must therefore be carefully discussed and examined with the person. It is advisable for families who want to and can provide financial assistance to their relative, to be cautious about how they do this. Giving large sums, or anything beyond a few dollars may not be a good idea. It might be more useful to purchase specific items, such as food or clothing, or to give checks that are made out to specific stores. While some people will still convert such assistance into money for drugs or alcohol, it can somewhat reduce the likelihood of this happening.

There are a variety of ways that family or caregivers can help a person manage their money. One option is having someone else assume complete control of a person's money. Another is having someone make sure rent and other essentials are paid before giving the person the remainder of their monthly income for spending money. Family members who become involved in helping manage a relative's finances run the risk of complicating their relationship with that person. It often works better to have a neutral third party—a county case manager or substitute payee—help in this area. Though objective outsiders may not be as involved with the person as we would like, they do allow family members to focus more on providing other kinds of emotional support. There is wisdom to the adage about not mixing business with other relationships.

Another common trigger of relapse with drugs and alcohol for people with a dual diagnosis is a recurrence or increase in the symptoms of their mental illness. Using drugs or alcohol will in turn decrease the effectiveness of medication and increase the psychiatric symptoms. For some, this happens very quickly. For others, it takes a little longer. It may be hard for an outside observer to know which came first. That, however, is not as important as getting a person the help needed, such as medication, talking to a therapist or counselor, or hospitalization. Trying to persuade the person to stop using drugs and alcohol might also help. If things get bad enough, this may not occur until the person winds up in a jail or hospital.

Often people receiving government benefits have more money at the beginning of the month, with which they can buy more coffee and cigarettes. It would be wise to notice whether this is when their symptoms increase. Nicotine and caffeine dilute the effects of most psychiatric medication. It is difficult, however, to continually adjust the dosage of medication needed to correspond to fluctuating use of such substances.

Random objective tests, such as urine toxicology screens, blood tests, or alcohol Breathalyzer tests, are tools that can be useful to people who want to avoid relapsing with substance use. Many programs use these. Some consumers in early recovery and family members initially have a negative reaction to the use of these tests. People in later stages of recovery, however, talk about how helpful these tests can be in maintaining sobriety. Random drug testing has stopped many people from acting on an impulse or craving to use. The knowledge that they may be found out is just enough added incentive for them to avoid using until they are able to do so on their own. A doctor, case manager, or family member can assist in arranging such tests and in reviewing the results.

The causes of relapse for mental illness must also be kept in mind. The following Quick Reference Guide outlines these.

LEADING CAUSES OF RELAPSE FOR MENTAL ILLNESS

- Predictable and unpredictable changes in severity of the illness.
- Prescribed medication is not effective enough.
- Not taking medication as prescribed.
- Using street drugs or alcohol.
- Using increased amounts of caffeine or nicotine.
- Increased level of stress (whatever the person experiences as stressful).
- Decreased level of social support.
- Significant changes in a person's routine or place of residence.

EARLY WARNING SIGNS

In chapter four some of the early warning signs of a psychiatric relapse were discussed. These are often idiosyncratic to each person. They usually include the beginning of symptoms the person experiences when ill, such as depression, mania, or psychosis. It is important for a person with co-occurring disorders and the members of their support system to also learn the early warning signs of relapse with substance use.

These may include some of the "addict behaviors" or drug-seeking behaviors described earlier. The person himself must begin to recognize the changes, often subtle, in thinking and feelings that occur. A person may begin having cravings or think more about drugs and alcohol. They may begin thinking about and missing their old "using buddies." Anger may be closer to the surface. Someone who regularly attends twelve-step meetings may stop going.

A good dual diagnosis or substance-abuse counselor or program will help each person to identify his or her unique early warning signs. These changes in thinking can be so subtle at first that they are almost unrecognizable to the person or those comprising their support system. Ideally, a person will, in time, be able to inform people who want to support them in living a clean, sober, and stable life, of their early warning signs. Support people will, in turn, be able to discuss any of these signs when they are noticed. It takes a good deal of time and experience to be able to recognize early warning signs of relapse for either substance abuse or serious mental illness.

INTERVENTIONS

The next important part of relapse prevention for either of the co-occurring disorders is developing interventions that a person can employ when early warning signs appear. This usually takes trial and error and involvement of support people. Following is a list of typical interventions that a person recovering from dual disorders and their caregivers would be wise to consider when symptoms, cravings, or other early warning signs occur. This is an expansion of the list offered on page 102.

- Contact a family member, friend, twelve-step sponsor, or someone with whom you can discuss your concerns. Brainstorm how to avoid using.
- Increase participation in spiritual activities, twelve-step meetings, or other support groups.

- Reduce contact with people who use, drink, or tell "war stories" (glorify) about using and drinking.
- Stay away from "slippery" places.
- Write about the changes in thinking or feeling.
- Meditate, or use other relaxation techniques.
- Take a bath.
- Do something you enjoy like going fishing, artwork, or playing music.
- Read spiritual, recovery, or inspirational material.
- Exercise.
- Use stress-reduction exercises.
- Clean your room or home.
- Revise the amount of structured activity in which you are involved.
- Review a list of the negative consequences of using.
- Have supportive people stay with you or hold your car keys or money.
- Whatever else you know that works.

EFFECTS OF MEDICATION AND STREET DRUGS

It is important for people with a dual diagnosis, their families, and caregivers to become familiar with the effects of drugs and alcohol and their interaction with psychiatric symptoms and medications prescribed to treat them. Most street drugs and alcohol will render psychiatric medication much less effective or even ineffective. They also generally increase a person's psychiatric symptoms. It is inadvisable for a person to take a dose of any medication when they are acutely intoxicated or under the influence of a large amount of street drugs. If, however, they have drunk or used a small or moderate amount, it is not dangerous to take many kinds of medications.

The effects of street drugs are usually divided into three general categories. There are drugs, including alcohol, which have a sedating or depressant effect, sometimes referred to as "downers." There are stimulants, or "uppers," which give people increased energy and decreased desire to sleep. The aftermath of each of these types of drugs produces the opposite effect of the drug itself. When people withdraw from prolonged use of an "upper," like "speed" (methamphetamine), they will be depressed. When "coming down" from "downers," like alcohol or opiates, they will feel agitated, anxious, and restless.

The third category of drugs includes ones that are chemically somewhat different from each other. What they have in common is that they produce "psychedelic" types of experiences. They are usually referred to as hallucinogens and produce effects similar to the symptoms of psychoses. They are likely to increase psychotic symptoms in people with schizophrenia, schizoaffective disorder, or other psychotic disorders. Drugs in this category include lysergic acid diethylamide (known on the street as acid or LSD), phencyclidine (known on the street as PCP or angel dust), and a drug similar to amphetamine that is known on the street as MDMA or Ecstasy. Stimulants may also increase psychotic symptoms.

Stimulants increase symptoms of mania, and depressants increase symptoms of depression. The opposite also holds some truth. "Uppers" may temporarily reduce symptoms of depression, and "downers" may temporarily reduce anxiety or symptoms of mania. Using these drugs to lessen symptoms, however, brings with it other problems. After stopping use of such drugs, symptoms will usually worsen.

Some medications can continue to be of value to people who are taking certain kinds of street drugs. For example, an antipsychotic medication will help a person with psychotic symptoms who takes a hallucinogen like LSD and becomes more psychotic, or has a "bad trip." The usual dose may not be as effective because their symptoms are worse, but it will not harm them.

On the other hand, some combinations of medications with alcohol or street drugs are potentially dangerous. The most lethal combination is mixing alcohol with antianxiety medications, such as Valium, Ativan, and Xanax. These, like alcohol, slow down the central nervous system. In combination, they can slow the respiratory system and heart enough to cause death.

The other potentially dangerous combinations involve mixing some kinds of antidepressant medications with certain street drugs or alcohol. The newer antidepressants, SSRIs (selective serotonin reuptake inhibitors), can be toxic if taken with stimulants or other drugs containing amphetamines, such as MDMA. An older category of antidepressants, monoamine oxidase (MAO) inhibitors, which are now infrequently prescribed, can be toxic if mixed with alcohol or stimulants.

Medications such as Artane and Cogentin, often prescribed to reduce side effects of antipsychotic medication, are generally not dangerous to take when someone has used street drugs or alcohol. Families should be aware, however, that these medications themselves are sometimes abused. They can be used to get "high" when not taken in conjunction with antipsychotic medication. Therefore, they should not be taken if the person is not taking their antipsychotic medication.

Thus, we see that the symptoms of psychiatric disorders are exactly the same as the effects produced by drugs and alcohol. The same effects also occur when the use of drugs and

Effects of Street Drugs and

Type of Street Drug	Symptoms/Effects	Withdrawal	Effects/Interaction with Antipsychotics
Downers/Sedatives Alcohol ―――――― Barbituates Painkillers Opiates Heroin	Sedation Slowed movements Slurred speech Confusion Glazed eyes Pinpoint pupils Lessens inhibitions Relief of anxiety	Anxiety Agitation Sweating Tremors	Increased sedation. Can slow breathing. May diminish or eliminate effects of medication.
Uppers/Stimulants Methamphetamine Cocaine ―――――― Caffeine Nicotine	Increased energy Decreased sleep Agitation Anxiety Dilated pupils Irritability	Depressed mood Irritability	May increase psychotic symptoms. Reduces effects of medication. Nicotine may reduce level of medication.
Hallucinogens PCP Mescaline LSD Psilocybin Ecstasy/Adam/ MDMA ―――――― Marijuana	Prominent hallucinations Agitation Dilated pupils	Most mild (some fatigue) to no effects Marijuana: insomnia, decreased appetite, irritability	Increases psychotic symptoms, thereby diminishing or eliminating effects of medication.

mpact on Psychiatric Medication

Effects/Interaction with Antidepressants	Effects/Interaction with Mood Stabilizers	Effects/Interaction with Antianxiety Medication
Alcohol with MAOIs can be dangerous. Others: Diminish effectiveness of medication.	Excessive alcohol use with lithium has potential for causing lithium toxicity, which can be dangerous.	Most dangerous combination. Slows central nervous system. Can cause death.
With SSRIs can be dangerous. May be fatal with MAOIs. Caffeine, Nicotine diminishes effectiveness.	Will generally diminish effectiveness of medication.	Counteracts effects of medication. May lead to cycle of alternately taking downers then uppers.
MDMA and SSRIs can be dangerous. MAOIs with MDMA can be fatal.	Will diminish effectiveness of medication.	With PCP can be dangerous due to incresed sedation. Slows breathing.

alcohol is stopped. If symptoms suddenly increase it is difficult to determine, without a urine or blood test, whether it is the illness or drug use at cause.

Some of the most important information about medications and drugs is offered in the Quick Reference Guide, Effects of Street Drugs and Impact on Psychiatric Medication. It provides a summary of the effects of each category of street drugs, followed by what happens when someone stops using them. Next are the interactions each category of street drugs has with each of the four major categories of psychiatric medication. The guide is not meant to be exhaustive but rather to alert readers as to which changes in a relative's behavior may indicate the use of certain drugs and what combinations are potentially dangerous.

Families and caregivers often wonder what to do if someone misses a dose of medication. Usually, the best thing for the person to do is to take the missed dose as soon as it is remembered and then take any remaining doses for that day at evenly spaced intervals. For example, if there are eight hours remaining in the day and two remaining doses, take them four hours apart. However, if a missed dose is remembered when it is almost time for the next scheduled dose, it is usually best to skip the missed dose. It is not usually advisable to double up on doses. Of course, it is always best to ask the prescribing physician specific questions about an individual's medication regime.

HELPING PEOPLE WHO DO NOT BELIEVE
THEY HAVE PROBLEMS

What can the support system of people with a dual diagnosis do to help? To a large extent this depends upon how much insight a person has into their disorders. Some people are aware that they have a dual diagnosis of both psychiatric and substance-use problems, while others do not believe that they have such problems despite all evidence to the contrary.

With those who do not believe they have one or both problems, it is best not to engage in endless arguments about that topic. Trying to convince someone who does not think they have a dual diagnosis that they have a mental illness and/or a serious substance-use problem is usually futile at best. At worst, it will cause serious distrust and damage to your relationship with the person. It is not necessary to agree with their view. It is advisable to be clear that you believe the person has these problems and would be better off getting help. If the person disagrees, it is wise to be respectful of their opinion and try to agree to disagree. The best strategy then is to focus on helping the person achieve their goals in life, maintaining as good a relationship as possible, safety, and the person's behavior.

If your loved ones do not accept that they are ill or have a substance-use problem, you would do best to use the suggestions made in chapter four about responding to delusions as a blueprint for your relationship with them. They may well have a delusional understanding of their symptoms. For instance, they may believe they are not able to work or do other things because there is a conspiracy preventing them.

The most effective strategy is to listen to their feelings, their pain, and concerns, without engaging in discussions of the delusional material. Let them know you understand how they feel, without confirming their understanding of why.

Empathize with the difficulties they are experiencing, such as having no friends or no work. Try to find any common ground, especially related to goals they have for their lives. Acknowledge shared concern about their well-being, their situation, your love for each other and family. The best any family member or professional can do to help improve the quality of consumers' lives is to focus on ways to support them in establishing and achieving the positive goals they have.

It is important to keep your expectations realistic; your loved ones may not be able to achieve all their goals. They may need help breaking them down into small realistic steps they can accomplish. They may also need to experience the natural consequences of their choices, such as not being able to get a job, before they are willing to consider getting some help or seeing a counselor. One thing to avoid is becoming a "nag," constantly focusing on what you think is wrong with them or what you think they should do.

Lack of insight into having a mental illness is one of the symptoms that some people with mental illness have. If this is true for your loved one, you are advised to read Xavier Amador's book entitled *I Am Not Sick, I Don't Need Help!* (2000, Vida Press). It provides an excellent discussion of research and practical advice for dealing with the problem of anosognosia, or lack of insight.

Similarly, people who abuse drugs and alcohol deny and minimize the extent of this problem. It is fine to tell the person that you think he is drinking or using. You may want to add that you are concerned about the negative consequences this may have, that you would hate to see them go through the pain of another hospitalization or stay in jail. Being more confrontational about substance use is appropriate.

It is important for families to set limits with relatives when they are in their addiction and behaving in unacceptable ways. People need to experience the negative consequences of such behaviors. It does no one any good in the long run to support or help bail out someone who is lying and stealing to get money or goods to sell for drugs and alcohol.

This can be difficult with a person who, at different times, exhibits symptoms of serious mental illness. When the mental illness is more acute, he or she needs more support and involvement from caregivers. Families and treatment providers have been struggling for years with this dilemma. It is a very complex art and skill to figure out when to be more "hardnosed," to set limits and deny requests for money or assistance that will be used to buy drugs or alcohol, and when to help someone suffering from a mental illness who could benefit from some additional support.

Treatment settings require that staff have familiarity with both types of problems and interventions, and know which tactic to use and when. For families unsure of which problem is more prominent at any one time, it is advisable to consult with professionals who are familiar with both psychiatric and substance-use disorders. Often one family member will advocate one approach, the "hard line" that is needed with substance abuse, while another family member will want to be more gentle and supportive. If everyone can understand that each approach is needed at different times, there may be fewer arguments. Remember that this is a very difficult assessment to make. Professionals working with a person frequently disagree on this very issue.

With people who do not accept that they have a dual diagnosis, many programs and services utilize a strategy known as "harm reduction." With this approach, the focus is on reducing the amount of harm that a person experiences as a result of their using, drinking, or having an untreated psychiatric disorder. This means that the provider does not refuse to work with the person or focus on trying to get a person to accept that they have problems and need help. Instead, the focus is on how people can live the best life possible and minimize the danger to which they expose themselves. This approach is an alternative to an "abstinence-based" substance-abuse program or service that requires participants to abstain from using drugs and alcohol. While abstinence is the long-term goal of a harm-reduction approach, it is not a requirement in the short run. The most important elements of a harm-reduction method are summarized in the following Quick Reference Guide:

This is how a harm-reduction approach would be applied to Tim, who has paranoid schizophrenia, smokes marijuana or drinks alcohol daily, and occasionally likes to "shoot" (in-

HOW TO HELP PEOPLE WHO DO NOT UNDERSTAND THAT THEY HAVE DUAL DISORDERS

- Develop a trusting relationship (listen, empathize, let them know you understand their perspective).
- Focus on their strengths, not weaknesses.
- Be positive, celebrate even the smallest success, avoid arguments.
- Help them attend to immediate needs (medical, food).
- Help them be as safe as possible.
- Try to minimize the harm resulting from use.
- Help them establish goals and ways to achieve them.
- Focus on their behavior and consequences vis-à-vis their goals.
- Be consistent.
- Keep your expectations realistic.

ject) heroin. Tim usually lives on the streets, or in a motel room when he has the money. He does not believe he has a mental illness or that his drug use is a problem. The focus with Tim would not be trying to get him to take psychiatric medication and go to a drug treatment program, though those might be big steps in the right direction. The focus instead would be to encourage Tim not to share needles with anyone when he shoots up, and to provide him with clean needles or bleach to clean his needles, so he will be less likely to contract the HIV virus or other contagious diseases. One might also talk with Tim about whether he would be interested in finding a doctor for his ear infection. Through helping Tim to address some of these needs or others that he identifies as problems, one might be able to begin building a relationship. At a later date, after sufficient trust has been established, it may be possible to discuss with Tim his substance use, psychiatric symptoms, or how he might improve his housing situation and achieve other goals.

AN INTERVENTION

Another approach sometimes used with people who are in denial of their substance use is a procedure known as doing "an intervention." When an intervention occurs, many people who are concerned about a person get together and confront the person. The person often does not know that this will be happening. A plan is developed ahead of time, often with a trained facilitator, as to where the person will be encouraged to get treatment. It can be very powerful to have a roomful of caring people—from various parts of a person's life—strongly and lovingly express concern, telling the person that he or she has a serious problem and needs help immediately.

Families often wonder if this is appropriate for someone with dual disorders. The answer highlights some of the ways treatment for such persons differs from treatment for people with a substance-abuse disorder alone. An intervention might be effective when used in a modified way, for some people with certain psychiatric disorders. It would depend in part on how acute their symptoms were at the time. Many people with schizophrenia or schizoaffective disorder would not be able to tolerate this kind of intervention. It could trigger or increase their symptoms. It would not be recommended for anyone who was having psychotic symptoms due to either drugs or a psychiatric disorder. It would be particularly inadvisable for someone with paranoid schizophrenia, as their delusions about people conspiring against them would very likely increase.

An intervention would have the best chance of success with a person who has a mood disorder, was currently psychiatrically stable, and relapsing in the use of drugs or alcohol.

HITTING BOTTOM

In the world of substance abuse and recovery, the concept of "hitting bottom" has been well established. "Hitting bottom" means that things become so bad for people that they are willing to consider making significant changes in their lives. It is often necessary for people to hit bottom before they can understand that they have a substance-use problem or a mental illness. Hitting bottom is a subjective experience and varies greatly from person to person. One person's "bottom" may resemble what someone else's life is like when things are relatively stable. Mary, for example, is a nurse who has done well in her career and takes medication for her bipolar disorder to keep that under control. She abuses medication that she gets prescribed by different doctors or steals from the clinic where she works. Before hitting bottom, she was not ready to accept the extent of her substance abuse. She lost her job, her nursing license, her relationship, her house, and was forced briefly to stay in a homeless shelter. That was Mary's "bottom."

Sue, on the other hand, has been homeless for years. She refused to take any psychiatric medication for her schizophrenia and used methamphetamine as often as she could. She was not willing to consider going to a treatment program until she was hospitalized, almost died during a bout of pneumonia, and her makeshift tent under a bridge was removed by the police. Only then did she agree to try living at a shelter and taking some medication. For Sue, this represents a major improvement in her life.

STAGES OF RECOVERY FROM SUBSTANCE USE FOR PEOPLE WHO UNDERSTAND THAT THEY HAVE A DUAL DIAGNOSIS

As public awareness of substance abuse and mental illness grows, more young people and families have the information and understanding to recognize warning signs of psychiatric disorders and substance abuse. Consequently, more people are obtaining treatment and services earlier on in the disorders. Early treatment increases the likelihood of a less severe illness and a better prognosis. As the stigma gradually decreases, people become less reluctant to seek the help they need. They are willing to participate in services described in chapter two. They make use of the new psychiatric medications available, some of which have minimal or no side effects for certain people. They also learn what it means to "work a program" of recovery from substance abuse.

Many people think that if an addict or alcoholic stops using drugs or alcohol then he or she is well on the road to recovery. More often, this is not the case. Certainly, abstaining from using is necessary to begin recovering from substance abuse. It is an enormous step to take. However, if this is all a person does, it is not likely to go very far. Someone who only stops using and makes no other change in his or her life is often referred to as a "dry drunk."

As discussed earlier, people who drink and use for a long time revolve much of their lives around drugs and alcohol. When they stop using, they need to learn how to deal with life, people, and problems in different ways. This is extremely difficult to do alone. Most people need the help of a counselor and a support program, such as Alcoholics Anonymous, to make the changes and learn the new skills necessary to build a new way of life. A "dry drunk" is much more likely to relapse and return to using than is someone in recovery who is "working a program." This is the term used for someone who is actively working a twelve-step program or another program of recovery from substance abuse. Such a person is learning different ways to handle relationships, responsibilities, cravings, feelings, and problems.

Recovery from substance abuse is a process that has several stages during which people typically address different issues. A very brief overview of the stages of recovery follows. It is recommended that families and people in recovery read more extensively about the process. *Staying Sober* by Terence Gorski and Merlene Miller (1986, Herald House/Independence Press) is one good place to find a more extensive description of this process for both addicts and alcoholics.

Early recovery lasts for at least the first year after one stops drinking or using. During this time, people may go through physical withdrawal from substances, depending upon how long and how much they have used. This can be extremely painful, frightening, and stressful. The best way to do this is under the care of a physician and a detoxification program. The most intense or acute part of a physical withdrawal usually lasts only a few days or a week at most. After that, a person experiences Post Acute Withdrawal Syndrome, or "PAWS." PAWS can last up to a year or more. During this time, a person may experience mood swings, irritability, memory problems, difficulty in thinking clearly, emotional over-reactions, emotional numbness, disturbances in sleep, hypersensitivity to stress, or difficulty in solving even relatively simple problems in life.

Addicts or alcoholics in early recovery are still a long way from feeling okay or feeling like "themselves." Those who began drinking or using in their teens have little sense of who they are as an adult. In early recovery, people go through a process of accepting that they have an addiction and recognizing the effects it has had on them physically, psychologically, and socially. They begin to learn or relearn what it is like to live and function without drugs or alcohol being the major focus. Families must not underestimate the enormity of such a transition. This is further complicated by a psychiatric disorder. People will likely experience more symptoms and need also to figure out how to manage them.

The process of recovery is always up and down. It does not happen smoothly, easily, and consistently. There are times when people feel stuck, discouraged, hopeless, have enormous cravings, and battle urges to return to old behaviors. It is then that family and caregivers can help by lovingly reminding them why they have undertaken this journey, and how much worse their lives would be if they again began to use or drink. It is useful to keep in mind a few of the most painful experiences people have had, such as living on the streets, being in jail, or prostituting to earn money for drugs. When struggling with the pain and agony of life without drugs, addicts and alcoholics are likely to forget the negative experiences of using until they learn different ways to cope.

DEVELOPING A HEALTHY LIFESTYLE

In the middle stages of recovery a person must learn to develop a well-balanced life. This is often a very new and different way of life. Due to the limitations of their mental illness and their substance use, people may not have experienced things others take for granted. For example, it is striking how many people with co-occurring disorders have no idea how to have fun without using. It can be a frightening experience for such people to go out into the world when they are clean and sober. Many have never celebrated a holiday or birthday without getting loaded. Many have never been sexual when they were not drinking or using.

Think of all the things that go into creating what you would consider a well-balanced life. These are all the things that people recovering from co-occurring disorders must learn how to include in the new lives they must build. The following is a daunting list of the many elements people must work on in the middle stages of recovery.

- Eating a balanced, healthy diet without large quantities of sugar and caffeine.
- Finding exercise they enjoy.
- Establishing healthy relationships with family and friends.
- Developing a spiritual practice.
- Finding productive activities, such as paid or volunteer work, school, hobbies.
- Learning to relax.

- Having fun.
- Practicing stress- and anger-management skills.
- Managing recurrences of psychiatric symptoms.
- Managing cravings for drugs and alcohol.
- Budgeting and managing money.

It is important that family and caregivers have patience while people are in the process of learning or relearning how to do all of the above. Some people will be working on this while experiencing psychiatric symptoms because the most effective combination of medication is still being determined.

In the later stages of recovery from substance abuse, a person integrates all that has been learned and practiced. They discover how to solve more complex problems in life and to modify areas of their lives that may not be working well. For people with more severe psychiatric symptoms, this too is more complicated. They must come to terms with the possibility that their capacity to do all that they would like may be limited by their illness.

HOW FAMILY AND CAREGIVERS CAN HELP

Research has shown that one of the best predictors of success for someone with co-occurring disorders is the presence of an empathic and hopeful, continuous relationship, where integrated treatment and coordination of care occurs through multiple treatment episodes. In order for this to occur, both a comprehensive, continuous, integrated system of care and individuals within that system who work with the person over time are needed.

Sometimes it is a case manager, doctor, or therapist who knows the person and continues to work with them through many ups, downs, relapses, and placements. Families often wind up doing this job because appropriate services are scant and, even where they exist, turnover among staff may be high. It is not an easy job for families or paid staff to perform. People with co-occurring disorders can be very difficult individuals with whom to work and maintain a relationship. Many of their behaviors are extremely off-putting, infuriating, and hurtful. Families often need to back away for periods of time to take care of themselves.

No matter how well-informed caregivers may be about substance-abuse and mental-illness recovery, there is a limit to how much they can do. If the person with the dual disorders does not meet you at least halfway, if he or she is not ready to make changes in his or her life, there is little anyone else can do. As much as people need help with recovery, unless they make some level of commitment to recover, no one else can do it for them. This is often a source of much frustration and pain for families who want so much to see the life of their loved one improve.

For most people, an extremely important aspect of recovery from substance abuse or mental illness is involvement with a community of people also in recovery. A twelve-step program is one very effective and accessible place to obtain this support. It is therefore useful for family and caregivers to become familiar with the principles and practices of twelve-step programs. One recommended way to do this is to attend several meetings. Many meetings are "open" to people who are not addicts or alcoholics. Experiencing meetings will provide a far broader understanding than reading about them. Below is a summary of many important aspects of twelve-step programs. It is offered to provide further insight into the minds of addicts and greater understanding of the changes that occur during the process of recovery.

Twelve-step programs offer much more than meetings.

They offer a community of people struggling with similar issues and supporting one another in many ways to stay clean and sober. There are clean-and-sober conventions, recreational activities, and social events. There is literature available to learn more about the concepts, philosophy, and new way of life often discussed. The philosophy is based upon many of the same core principles taught by most religions. Being a productive member of a community, living an honest life, respecting oneself and others are promoted. People are encouraged to think about their behavior, take responsibility for mistakes, and make amends to those they have hurt.

The following is a list of slogans and phrases frequently used as reminders for concepts and values central to the twelve-step culture. There are also brief descriptions or explanations of the tendencies of addicts they are meant to address.

- "One Day at a Time" (Try to stay clean and sober just for today. Do not focus too far into the future.)
- "Easy Does It" (Take things at a slower, more manageable pace.)
- "Progress Not Perfection" (Focus on gradually doing a little better. Relax perfectionist standards.)
- "Keep It Simple" (Do not make things too complicated to handle.)
- "First Things First" (Focus on here-and-now priorities instead of anxiety about possible future problems.)
- "Stinkin' Thinkin'" (Do not rationalize drinking, using, and addict behaviors.)
- "Turn It Over" (Let a power greater than us take care of some things. We cannot control everything.)
- "Taking an Inventory" (Recognize mistakes we have made and how we have hurt others because of our ad-

dictions. Each person is encouraged to take only his or her own inventory.)

- "Making Amends" (Acknowledge our mistakes and ask forgiveness from those we have hurt because of our addiction.)
- "Fake It 'til You Make It" (Do or say the right or healthy thing even when we feel like doing otherwise.)
- "Pulling a Geographic" (Move or change place of work or residence believing that this will change how we feel. Running away from problems.)
- "Giving Back" (Offer individuals or the community some of what we have learned and has been given to us.)
- "Walk the Talk" (Practice what we preach. Unlike those who merely "talk the talk.")
- "Doing 90 in 90" (Attend 90 meetings in 90 days to re-focus on recovery after relapsing, or as intervention to avoid an impending relapse.)

Working a twelve-step program also entails having one or more "sponsors." Getting a sponsor is a significant benchmark and a very important part of working a program. Sponsors have been working a program of recovery for a while and help guide their "sponsee" through the process of "working the steps." This usually involves writing and discussing each of the twelve steps as it applies very personally to the sponsee. Sponsors are also available to talk to their sponsees if they are having a hard time or feel like drinking or using. Sponsors are not counselors or therapists but people who can listen, share their own personal experience in similar situations, and help others think of healthy alternatives to using. It is essential that people looking for a sponsor find someone with whom they feel comfortable talking, someone they respect, and from whom they can learn. Participating in twelve-step meetings provides a place for people to do what is said in almost every meeting: to share experience, strength, and hope to solve common problems.

There are several questions that often arise about twelve-step meetings for people with co-occurring disorders. The first has to do with how well people who attend meetings understand psychiatric symptoms and medication. This varies enormously from meeting to meeting. Anyone who wants to get involved in meetings is encouraged to try out several meetings until he or she finds a group with which he or she feels comfortable. Some groups tend to have older participants, some younger, some all women, some only alcoholics, some addicted to other drugs, and so forth. While the national office of Alcoholics Anonymous takes few "official positions," they have condoned the taking of psychiatric medication for those people who have it appropriately prescribed. Although not all people who attend meetings are aware of this, an increasing number of participants are. There are still some who incorrectly believe that people in recovery from drugs or alcohol should not take any kind of medication regardless of what other illnesses they may have. It can be very difficult for people with a dual diagnosis to encounter such views, especially early in their recovery. Those more solid in themselves and their recovery are able to educate twelve-step participants who espouse such mistaken ideas.

There is a growing movement that affords people with co-occurring disorders a wonderful alternative to traditional twelve-step meetings. These are twelve-step groups specifically designed for people with a dual diagnosis. A group called Dual Recovery Anonymous (DRA), for instance, has done a brilliant job of modifying the twelve steps to make them more relevant and supportive to people with co-occurring psychiatric disorders. It would be wise for anyone interested in attending twelve-step meetings to look for such a group in your area or to consider forming one. There are also readings and other materials available that might interest family, caregivers, and people with a dual diagnosis who do not want to attend meetings. Such information can be obtained online at the DRA website: *www.draonline.org*, or by calling the DRA World Services Central Office at 1-877-883-2332.

Another issue that can be a stumbling block for people with dual disorders or their caregivers is the "God language" used in traditional twelve-step literature. What many people do not realize is that it is perfectly acceptable to think of any kind of "higher power" in place of a more traditional notion of God. While twelve-step programs do encourage people to develop spirituality and to use meditation, they do not insist on any particular belief in God. People can very effectively work the steps by thinking of some force greater than that which compels them to use or drink. It can be an external force such as nature or an internal one such as a "higher self." There are other recovery meetings, such as Rational Recovery, where there are no references to God while supporting people to live clean and sober lives. These may be more appropriate for people whose psychiatric symptoms include religious delusions or preoccupation. As with DRA, these unfortunately are not yet available in all areas.

It behooves families to support any efforts individuals make toward finding a support group with which they feel comfortable. There are twelve-step groups geared toward particular drug use, such as Narcotics Anonymous (NA) or Marijuana Users Anonymous (MA). It is not particularly important what a person's substance of abuse was. What is most important is finding a group of people with whom a person is comfortable talking about recovery, and receiving and giving support.

There are several other crucial ways in which family and caregivers can support someone with a dual diagnosis to have the best life possible. They are summarized in the Quick Reference Guide entitled How Families Can Help Minimize Substance Abuse.

Families and caregivers who want fully to support someone in not using and drinking do not use or drink around the person. They also do not keep alcohol or drugs readily accessible to the person. Some argue that the person will have to get used to being around alcohol, that it is his or her problem, and that others should not have to change their behaviors. This is similar to blowing smoke in the face of someone with emphysema who is trying to quit smoking. Yes, people in recovery will see drugs and alcohol used almost everywhere they turn in most cultures. This is precisely the reason those who love them will provide them with a safe haven. What people in recovery need are others who can model how to celebrate, have fun, and socialize without drugs and alcohol. For some consumers, it is hard to find family and friends willing to do this.

If refraining from drinking or using around a relative or friend in recovery seems too large a burden, it is usually an indicator that you too have a problem with drugs or alcohol. People who do not have any problem with alcohol do not feel it is much of a sacrifice to forgo that glass of beer, or wine with dinner, or cocktail before dinner. If this issue stirs strong feelings, you are urged to examine your own relationship to alcohol and drugs. As discussed earlier, one of the leading relapse triggers is being around "slippery people." When a family routinely uses alcohol or drugs, this poses a special dilemma for people in recovery who also want to stay connected to their family. Sometimes it means having to make an extraordinarily difficult choice between continuing contact with family or staying clean, sober, and stable.

HOW FAMILIES CAN HELP
MINIMIZE SUBSTANCE ABUSE

- Talk about concerns despite relative's denial.
- Educate yourself.
- Recognize the magnitude of the undertaking of stopping use of drugs or alcohol.
- Learn about the interactions of drugs and alcohol with symptoms and medication.
- Encourage treatment and support groups (DRA, AA, Rational Recovery).
- Encourage any nondelusional spiritual practice that provides comfort.
- Keep clear limits and boundaries.
- Do not enable or support the use of drugs or alcohol.

FAMILY RECOVERY

We have addressed what recovery from mental illness means to those surviving psychiatric symptoms. We have discussed recovery from substance abuse as well. Now let us look at the recovery process that family members experience.

When a family member experiences the transformation that occurs with a mental illness and a substance-use disorder, the family experiences a trauma of its own. There is a process of recovering from that trauma that each and every family member also experiences. This entails readjusting our attitudes, feelings, beliefs, and perceptions about ourselves, our family

- Tolerate relapses but distinguish from resuming a pattern of using.
- In times of stress, if asked, remind your relative of healthy alternatives to using.
- Connect negative consequences with use.
- Do not try to control the person.
- Do not drink or use around your relative.
- Do not keep alcohol or drugs available.
- Participate in family support groups, like ALANON, CoDA, NAMI.
- Do not blame or feel ashamed of yourself.
- Do not isolate yourself.
- Develop a plan for yourselves, what you will do in case of emergency, **if possible** include the ill person.
- Get help for siblings who often get lost in all the focus given to the consumer.

members, and about life. It is natural to have strong reactions to intense, painful, or traumatic experiences. By moving through those feelings, we undergo a process of self-renewal that transforms us. While it can shake us to our core, we often emerge stronger and more connected to who we really are, to those closest to us, and to what is most important to us.

There are several things about this process that family and caregivers should keep in mind. As with any recovery process, each person goes at her or his own pace. It affects different family members in somewhat different ways. It is not a linear process. There will be movement in and among the different stages.

Often the first stage is denial or disbelief that mental ill-ness or substance abuse could be happening in our family, to our loved one. This is a natural reaction to hearing any sort of shocking news, especially a diagnosis of serious illness. All family members and professionals must learn to accept that some denial will occur. Compassion and empathy are the best response. What is best to reflect back to a person in this stage is an understanding of how hard it is to accept that the changes or disorders are occurring.

Gradually people come to recognize that the problems are real and not going to be quickly resolved. They may begin to feel guilt, shame, the loss of the person, and of their own life as it had previously been. As people go through this stage, others can assist by labeling the grieving process as such and acknowledging the feelings that are occurring. It is also help-ful to discuss the crises in faith that may occur. People may well question all spiritual beliefs and ideas about any mean-ing and order that exists in life.

As these feelings are processed, the desire to cope and re-gain a sense of competence comes to the foreground. People focus more on finding solutions and effective interventions. Professionals and others can now be most helpful by provid-ing education, information about the disorders, services and treatments available, and coping strategies. Frustration, anger, and discouragement about the lack of adequate services might surface at this time or whenever families are confronted with these painful realities. Professionals would be wise to try not to take such feelings personally, but to focus instead on how all participants can work together to help the consumer make the most of available resources.

Over time, everyone involved can experience a greater sense of confidence and ability to cope with the myriad issues they face. People are able to move through the process to a new level of awareness about themselves, their relative, and the services system. Though symptoms may remain, families are able to let go of most of the guilt and shame and to focus increasingly on how best to adapt. They have a better sense of realistic expectations for themselves, their relative, and professionals. They may turn some of their energy toward political advocacy, making changes in local services' delivery systems, or helping other families to cope. They find new ways to live with and accept the changes in their loved one and in the family. They are again able to better enjoy other people and activities in their lives.

Some people, however, have great difficulty in getting through this process. They may need individual counseling and ongoing group support. They may be stuck in one stage of their recovery or struggling with issues of co-dependence.

CO-ADDICTION OR CO-DEPENDENCE

When a family member has a serious disorder, it is natural for family and friends to want to help. Most parents or primary caretakers want to do whatever they can to make the person feel better. Family members are often willing to devote a good deal of time, energy, and resources to helping someone in crisis. There is nothing wrong with this. Problems arise when the crises become continuous and the caregiver devotes so much time and energy to the consumer that helping becomes the sole focus of the caregiver's life. Helping the person in need begins to consume the caregiver's thoughts and behaviors in the same way that drugs and alcohol consume an addict. This is sometimes called "co-dependence." Because that term has developed negative connotations for some people, the term "co-addiction" is used instead. Co-addiction is defined as a condition in which life has become unmanageable as a result of being closely involved with a person with a serious mental illness or a dual diagnosis. One possible indicator of co-addiction is having trusted friends or relatives suggest that you are overly involved with your family member.

Co-addiction follows a predictable progression. It gets worse over time unless a person becomes aware of the problem and takes specific steps to ameliorate it. As with addiction, it can become a chronic problem prone to recurrence (relapse). People must learn how to counteract co-addiction and obtain appropriate support for doing so. For some, this is best done with the help of an individual psychotherapist or counselor. For others, attending a support group works best. As with recovery from addiction or mental illness, it is ex-

---

CO-ADDICTION

Progression of Co-addiction:

1. Early stage—Try to help; devote time, energy, and financial aid to relative in need.
2. Middle stage—Try harder; efforts to help feel more desperate and intense.
   - Feel extremely protective and preoccupied with well-being of relative.
   - Engage in fewer activities that nurture you.
3. Later stage—Family collapse or disintegration is evidenced by any or all of the following:
   - Specific, repetitive patterns of self-defeating or ineffective behaviors.
   - Thinking and behavior is out of control.
   - Stress-related illnesses appear.

tremely difficult for a person to successfully recover entirely on his or her own.

Just as addiction and recovery have various stages, so does co-addiction. The Quick Reference Guide entitled Co-Addiction summarizes the stages of co-addiction and recovery from it.

Some families of people with psychiatric disorders have been very put off and offended by support groups for co-addiction, such as Co-dependents Anonymous (CODA) or Al-Anon. Others have found them very useful. It is best for people who think they may have problems in this area to at-

---

- The physical, social, and psychological well-being of family members significantly deteriorates.

Recovery from Co-addiction Requires:

- Learning to accept and detach from the symptoms of addiction and mental illness.
- Learning to manage and control the symptoms of co-addiction.
- Choosing appropriate behaviors, such as those outlined on pages 138–139 (Keeping a Life of Your Own).
- Learning to manage relapses to co-addictive behaviors.
- Maintaining a healthy lifestyle, including getting support for co-addiction and involvement with people and activities that have nothing to do with the person with a dual diagnosis.

tend one of these meetings and see if it is useful. What would be most helpful for families who have a relative with co-occurring disorders is a support group for precisely such families. Those active in NAMI are encouraged to establish local dual-diagnosis family support groups.

Families of people with co-occurring disorders are faced with the extraordinary challenge of learning how to vary the amount and type of involvement to offer, as the severity of psychiatric symptoms and substance abuse varies in their relative. When psychiatric symptoms become acute, more support and family involvement is often appropriate. When people begin using or drinking, a more confrontational approach is called for. When people are actively using, drinking, and engaging in addict behaviors, there may be little anyone can do to get them to stop. The approach that makes the most sense then is to keep enough distance to protect yourself and others from theft and verbal, physical, financial, or other forms of abuse. Contact might be limited to determining if they require an emergency intervention, such as calling the police or helping to arrange a hospitalization.

Most twelve-step meetings end with the Serenity Prayer. This wisdom is useful for all people, especially those with co-occurring disorders, their friends, and family. It is offered here as a reminder of one of the most important coping strategies for all. Sometimes "Lord" is the first word. It works as well to think of any form of higher power or the source of all life and wisdom. From that source we ask to be granted the serenity to accept the things we cannot change, the courage to change the things we can, and the wisdom to know the difference.

Appendix: Medications

THE INFORMATION OFFERED HERE is intended as a guide for families, friends, and patients. It is by no means exhaustive. It does not include all medications used or all possible side effects. It is offered in order to familiarize the reader with many of the medications most commonly used to treat serious mental illnesses, and with their common side effects. It is not a substitute for the direction of a personal physician. *All prescribed medications should be taken only under the supervision of a physician. It is unwise to vary the dose of these medications or to abruptly stop taking them without consulting a doctor.* Some of the side effects are likely to increase with an abrupt change in dosage.

Medications are complicated; some are grouped by their chemical makeup. For example, among the antidepressants we can differentiate the tricyclics and the selective serotonin reuptake inhibitors (SSRIs). Those that are more similar chemically tend to have similar side effects. No one medication is likely to produce all the side effects listed here, and no one person is likely to experience all the side effects listed under each category. Many people experience few side effects to psychiatric medications, or none at all. Side effects or reactions should be reported to your doctor.

The most effective dosage for any individual needs to be determined over time and is dependent on age, size, ethnicity, severity of symptoms, and the person's response to the medication. The dosages listed here are in milligrams and represent the usual outpatient dose. For inpatients and emergencies, higher doses are often used on a short-term basis.

If your relative's prescribed medication dosage is different than what is listed here, speak with the doctor. There could be a good reason that a less common medication or dose is indicated. To learn more about these medications, consult one of the books listed in the Resource Directory, which follows.

The time it takes for therapeutic effects to occur varies. With certain medications (antiparkinsonians, antianxiety medications, sleeping pills, and antipsychotics), some effects may be felt within an hour. For antidepressants and some medication for bipolar disorder, it usually takes about two weeks for any effect to occur, and it may take up to six weeks before the full therapeutic effect is felt.

There is also great variation in the length of time medications remain in the body. Some wear off within a few hours, while others may continue to produce a therapeutic effect for days after use has been discontinued.

MOST COMMON BRAND NAME	GENERIC NAME	RANGE OF OUTPATIENT DAILY DOSE (MG)	THERAPEUTIC EFFECTS	POSSIBLE SIDE EFFECTS
ATYPICAL (newer) ANTIPSYCHOTIC MEDICATION				
Clozaril	Clozapine	200–900	Reduces psychotic symptoms and reduces negative symptoms of schizophrenia (e.g., lack of motivation)	Agranulocytosis (requires weekly blood test to monitor), drowsiness, drooling, dizziness, headache, low blood pressure, weight gain, increased cholesterol, increased blood sugar.
Risperdal	Risperidone	.05–8	Same as above	Sedation, nausea, constipation, shakiness, muscle stiffness, sexual dysfunction, menstrual irregularities, some weight gain, increased cholesterol, increased blood sugar.
Zyprexa	Olanzapine	5–20	Same as above	Sedation, weight gain, increased cholesterol, increased blood sugar.
Seroquel	Quetiapine Fumarate	300–800	Same as above	Sedation, some weight gain, headache, dizziness, constipation, dry mouth, increased cholesterol, increased blood sugar.

MOST COMMON BRAND NAME	GENERIC NAME	RANGE OF OUTPATIENT DAILY DOSE (MG)	THERAPEUTIC EFFECTS	POSSIBLE SIDE EFFECTS
ATYPICAL (newer) ANTIPSYCHOTIC MEDICATION (*cont.*)				
Geodon	Ziprasidone	80–160	Same as above	Anxiety, upset stomach, weakness, constipation, diarrhea, dry mouth, loss of appetite, muscle pain, restlessness, increased cholesterol, increased blood sugar. Can cause heart irregularities when taken with certain medication, including Mellaril.
Abilify	Aripiprazole	10–30	Same as above	Anxiety, headache, insomnia, nausea, lightheadedness.

Compared to traditional antipsychotics, all of the above have much lower risk of Parkinson-like, extrapyramidal symptoms (EPS), such as tremors, muscle stiffness or rigidity, restlessness, and lack of facial expression, and a lower risk of tardive dyskinesia, sometimes irreversible abnormal movements, most commonly of tongue and mouth.

MOST COMMON BRAND NAME	GENERIC NAME	RANGE OF OUTPATIENT DAILY DOSE (MG)	THERAPEUTIC EFFECTS	POSSIBLE SIDE EFFECTS
TRADITIONAL ANTIPSYCHOTIC MEDICATION (Major Tranquilizers)				
Prolixin Prolixin decanoate (long-acting injection)	Fluphenazine	5–60 12.5–100 every 2–4 weeks	Relieves symptoms of psychosis such as: hallucinations, delusions, and confused thinking. Also improves concentration and reduces anxiety and agitation.	More common: Drowsiness, dry mouth, constipation, difficulty urinating, blurry vision, restlessness, tremors, muscle stiffness, dizziness (low blood pressure), sun sensitivity, decreased movement, weight gain. Less common: Loss of menstrual periods and sex drive, lactation.
Haldol Haldol decanoate (long-acting injection)	Haloperidol	2–30 25–200 once a month		

Less Common Brand Names (generic names) and doses:
Thorazine (Chlorpromazine) 100–800, Mellaril (Thioridazine) 100–600, Trilafon (Perphenazine) 8–64, Stelazine (Trifluoperazine) 5–40, Navane (Thiothixene) 5–30, Serentil (Mesoridazine) 100–400, Loxitane (Loxapine) 60–250

SIDE EFFECT MEDICATION (Antiparkinsonian)				
Cogentin Artane Akineton Kemadrin Benadryl	Benztropine Trihexyphenidyl Biperiden Procyclidine Diphenhydramine	1–8 1–15 1–8 7.5–20 25–100	Reduces: stiff muscles, tremors, restlessness, shuffling walk, lack of facial expression, drooling, eyes "stuck" in upward glance.	Dry mouth, constipation, blurry vision, drowsiness, nausea.

MOST COMMON BRAND NAME	GENERIC NAME	RANGE OF OUTPATIENT DAILY DOSE (MG)	THERAPEUTIC EFFECTS	POSSIBLE SIDE EFFECTS
ANTIDEPRESSANT MEDICATION **Selective Serotonin Reuptake Inhibitors (SSRIs)**				
Prozac Paxil Zoloft Luvox Celexa Lexapro	Fluoxetine Parotexine Sertraline Fluvoxamine Citalopram Escitalopram	10–80 20–50 50–200 50–300 40–60 10–20	Reduces: depression, lethargy, chronic fatigue.	Dizziness, increased sweating, blurry vision, sun sensitivity, weight gain, difficulty sleeping, nausea, vomiting, insomnia, headache, agitation, sexual dysfunction.
Tricyclics				
Elavil or Endep Norpramin Tofranil Aventyl or Pamelor Vivactil Sinequan or Adapin	Amitriptyline Desipramine Imipramine Nortriptyline Protriptyline Doxepin	75–150 75–200 30–200 30–150 10–60 25–300	Same as above	Sedation, dizziness, increased blood pressure, blurry vision, weight gain, sun sensitivity, rapid heartbeat.
Chemically Different from Tricyclics or SSRIs				
Wellbutrin Wellbutrin-SR (sustained release = slow acting)	Bupropion	150–450 150–300	Same as above	Agitation, dry mouth, insomnia, headache, rash, constipation, tremor, nausea.

MOST COMMON BRAND NAME	GENERIC NAME	RANGE OF OUTPATIENT DAILY DOSE (MG)	THERAPEUTIC EFFECTS	POSSIBLE SIDE EFFECTS
ANTIDEPRESSANT MEDICATION (*cont.*) Chemically Different from Tricyclics or SSRIs:				
Desyrel	Trazodone	50–400	Same as above	Dry mouth, dizziness, nausea, drowsiness, headache, musculoskeletal pain. Rare: painful sustained erection.
Serzone	Nefazodone	200–600	Same as above	Sedation, nausea, vomiting, headache, dizziness. Less common: liver problems.
Remeron	Mirtazapine	15–60	Same as above	Sedation, weight gain, dry mouth, dizziness.
Effexor Effexor-XR (slow release)	Venlafaxine	75–375	Same as above	Similar to SSRIs, and may increase blood pressure.

Monoamine oxidase inhibitors (MAOIs) such as Marplan (Isocarboxazid), Nardil (Phenelzine), and Parnate (Tranylcypromine) are rarely used anymore due to the necessary dietary restrictions.

MOST COMMON BRAND NAME	GENERIC NAME	RANGE OF OUTPATIENT DAILY DOSE (MG)	THERAPEUTIC EFFECTS	POSSIBLE SIDE EFFECTS
MEDICATION FOR BIPOLAR DISORDER (MOOD STABILIZERS)				
Depakote	Divalproex Sodium	500–3000	Helps even out both manic and depressive mood swings.	Nausea, fatigue, indigestion, diarrhea, skin rash, vomiting, dizziness, muscle ache, weight gain, constipation, pancreatitis, appetite loss, liver problems, birth defects if taken during pregnancy.
Eskalith, or Lithane, or Lithobid, or Lithonate, or Lithotabs	Lithium	600–1,800	Same as above	Upset stomach, nausea, diarrhea, vomiting, acne, hand tremors, weight gain, birth defects if taken during pregnancy, hypo (low) thyroid, increased frequency of urination, fatigue, metallic taste in mouth.
Tegretol	Carbamazepine	400–1600	Reduces mood swings. Usually taken with lithium or Depakote. Sometimes taken alone.	Sedation, dizziness, loss of balance, vision changes, nausea, vomiting, blood disorders, irregular heartbeat, rash, liver problems, birth defects if taken during pregnancy.

MOST COMMON BRAND NAME	GENERIC NAME	RANGE OF OUTPATIENT DAILY DOSE (MG)	THERAPEUTIC EFFECTS	POSSIBLE SIDE EFFECTS
MOOD STABLIZERS (*cont.*)				
Neurontin	Gabapentin	300–3600	Same as above (Also used for anxiety and chronic pain.)	Sedation, dizziness, vision changes, loss of balance.
Topamax	Topiramate	100–400	Same as above Usually taken with other mood stabilizers.	Psychomotor slowing, difficulty with concentration, confusion, weakness, somnolence, dizziness, memory loss, weight loss, tremor, vision changes, loss of balance. Rare: kidney stones.
Lamictal	Lamotrigine	50–500	Same as above Effective in preventing bipolar depression.	Dizziness, sedation, headache, vision changes, loss of balance, nausea, weight gain, severe rash.

MOST COMMON BRAND NAME	GENERIC NAME	RANGE OF OUTPATIENT DAILY DOSE (MG)	THERAPEUTIC EFFECTS	POSSIBLE SIDE EFFECTS
ANTIANXIETY MEDICATION (Minor Tranquilizers)				
Valium Librium Serax Tranxene Ativan Xanax Klonopin	Diazepam Chlordiazepoxide Oxazepam Clorazepate Lorazepam Alprazolam Clonazepam	5–40 5–100 30–120 7.5–60 1–6 1–10 .5–4	Reduces anxiety.	Psychological and/or physical dependence, withdrawal symptoms when drug stopped, increases effects of drinking alchol, drowsiness, morning hangover, gastro-intestinal distress, lack of coordination.
Less common brand names: Centrax, Paxipam, Equanil, Miltown.				
Chemically Different				
BuSpar	Buspirone	20–60	Same as above	Nonaddictive. Nausea, headache, restlessness.
HYPNOTICS (Sleeping Pills)				
Dalmane Restoril Halcion Desyrel Ambien	Flurazepam Temazepam Triazolam Trazodone Zolpidem	15–30 15–30 .125–.25 25–100 5–10	Relieves insomnia.	Same as minor tranquilizers
Chemically Different				
Benadryl	Diphenhydramine	25–50	Sedating antihistamine	Dry mouth, persistent drowsiness, difficulty concentrating. Nonaddictive.

Some antianxiety medication listed above and some antidepressant medication, such as Trazodone and Elavil, may be prescribed in lower doses to help with sleep problems.

Resource Directory

THROUGHOUT THE BOOK WE have emphasized that families and friends of people with mental illness need support and education in order to deal effectively with their situation. Listed here are some of the resources that are available to you. While you need not look into all the options available, please pursue some. As noted throughout the book, the most important resource is NAMI (formerly National Alliance for the Mentally Ill). If you do nothing else, you would be wise to get on the mailing list of your local (and preferably state and national) chapter, usually referred to as an affiliate. It would be best to attend a meeting so you can meet others in similar situations. You will also then know where to turn when specific questions or crises arise.

If you cannot find your local chapter of NAMI listed in the telephone directory, call the national office at (703) 524-7600. They will be happy to send you information about support groups in your area. NAMI operates a toll-free HelpLine: 1-800-950-NAMI. An enormous amount of information is available on the NAMI website: *www.NAMI.org*. NAMI has also organized a free twelve-week course for family caregivers of individuals with severe mental illnesses. Taught by trained family members, it is called the Family-to-Family Education Program. All instruction and course materials are free and can be obtained through NAMI. This course has been extremely helpful to families throughout the United States.

If you are interested in buying any of the books listed below, you may first want to check with NAMI as it has some of them available at a discounted price. You can call the NAMI HelpLine and request a current *NAMI Resource Catalog*, order online at the NAMI website, or try other online booksellers. It is quite possible that your local NAMI affiliate has a library where you can borrow books and tapes on mental illness that may not be available in public libraries. Some of the videotapes listed can be ordered through the Mental Illness Education Project.

Ask your local bookstore to order any books they do not have in stock. You can similarly request that your local library order books or tapes they do not have. This serves the additional purpose of making the material more readily available to others in need.

What follows is only a partial list of the books, journals, websites, and videos now available about mental illness. They will provide you with a starting point. As you begin to explore these resources you will find out about others. You can decide how much or how little you want to read, hear, see, and discuss about mental illness. There is a wide range of material available both in terms of media (books, videos, and so forth) and the style of presentation. Some are factual while others offer more personal accounts. There are shorter works written for the average person, lengthier ones written for professionals, and everything in between. Choose those that best suit you.

Schizophrenia

Surviving Schizophrenia: A Manual for Families, Consumers, and Providers, Fourth Edition by E. Fuller Torrey, M.D. (Harper-Collins, 2001). Written by an authority in the field of schizophrenia, who has a sister with schizophrenia. Considered the bible by many families with a relative who has schizophrenia, it is packed with useful information.

Schizophrenia: Straight Talk for Families and Friends by Maryellen Walsh (Warner Books, 1986). Written by a parent who, as a professional writer, thoroughly researched the field. The book is emotional, touching, full of understanding and some practical advice, and written with a sense of humor.

Coping with Schizophrenia: A Guide for Families by Kim Mueser, Ph.D., and Susan Gingerich, M.S.W. (New Harbinger, 1994). Many useful worksheets and practical suggestions. Especially useful for families with a relative who has schizophrenia and is living at home.

Bipolar Disorder and Depression

The Depression Workbook: A Guide for Living with Depression and Manic Depression, Second Edition by Mary Ellen Copeland, M.S. (New Harbinger, 2002). Provides a brief overview of symptoms, other issues consumers face, and treatments; then focuses on excellent self-help strategies for coping with mood disorders.

The Depression Sourcebook by Brian Quinn, Ph.D. (McGraw-Hill, 2000). A good basic guide to understanding mood disorders, how to alleviate symptoms and understand causes. This revised second edition provides new information on psychotherapy, bipolar disorders, depression in children and elderly people, medications, and treatment options such as exercise and nutrition.

When Someone You Love Is Depressed: How to Help Your Loved One Without Losing Yourself by Laura Rosen, Ph.D., and Xavier Amador, Ph.D. (Fireside Press, 1996). Focusing on family members, in particular partners, it offers ways to minimize the negative impact depression can have on close relationships.

What to Do When Someone You Love Is Depressed by Mitch Golant, Ph.D., and Susan K. Golant. (Henry Holt, 1996). A compassionately written discussion of how to recognize and best handle depression in a loved one. It is especially recommended for families newly dealing with depression. It includes examples of reactions family members experience and myths about mental illness.

Mental Illnesses in General

I Am Not Sick, I Don't Need Help! by Xavier Amador, Ph.D. (Vida Press, 2000). An excellent book. The first to address, in both a scientific and practical way, the problem of lack of insight into mental illness. Compassion and instructions are provided for families with a relative who does not understand that he or she has an illness and needs treatment.

The Burden of Sympathy: How Families Cope with Mental Illness by David Karp (Oxford University Press, 2000). Written by a sociology professor who also suffers from severe depression. Based on interviews with sixty families, the book captures the essence of caring and caregivers for families of people with serious mental illness.

The Caring Family: Living with Chronic Mental Illness by Kayla Bernheim, Richard Lewine, and Caroline Beale (Random House, 1982). Does not describe or differentiate specific types of illnesses, but gives good advice to families regarding the feelings and practical problems resulting from having a relative with a severe and persistent mental illness.

The Broken Brain: The Biological Revolution in Psychiatry by Nancy C. Andreasen, M.D. (Harper & Row, 1984). Provides a very readable discussion of the biomedical aspect of serious mental illnesses, including a description of how the brain works.

Medications

The Essential Guide to Psychiatric Drugs, Third Edition by Jack M. Gorman, M.D. (St. Martin's Press, 1997). This is an excellent reference book. It offers both a general discussion of psychiatric drugs and basic information about most medications used for depression, anxiety, bipolar disorder, schizophrenia, sleep disorders, and substance abuse.

Consumer's Guide to Psychiatric Drugs by John Preston, Psy.D., John O'Neal, M.D., and Mary Talaga, R.Ph. (New Harbinger, 2000). Another good reference book that provides both general issues related to taking medication, as well as extensive descriptions of many psychiatric medications and some "nonpharmaceutical approaches."

For Siblings and Offspring

My Sister's Keeper: Learning to Cope with a Sibling's Mental Illness by Margaret Moorman (Norton, 1992). A most insightful description of the effects of mental illness on a family and a sibling's eventual acceptance.

The Four of Us: A Family Memoir by Elizabeth Swados (Farrar, Straus, & Giroux, 1991). An extensive account of the impact of mental illness on a sibling, as well as on parents.

Troubled Journey: Coming to Terms with the Mental Illness of a Sibling or Parent by Diane I. Marsh, Ph.D., and Rex M. Dickens (Tarcher/Putnam, 1997). A blend of theoretical understanding and heartfelt compassion for siblings and offspring.

He Was Still My Daddy: Coming to Terms with Mental Illness by Laurie Samsel Olson (Ogden House, 1994). A very poignant, personal, and frank description of what it is like growing up with a father who developed paranoid schizophrenia.

The Invulnerable Child by E. James Anthony and Bertram J. Cohler (Guilford Press, 1987). An in-depth exploration of the impact on a child of being raised by a psychotic parent. The child's development of a seemingly well-adjusted "invulnerable" facade is well described.

The Girl with the Crazy Brother by Betty Hyland (Franklin Watts, 1987). A very enjoyable, readable story written for young readers, about a high school student torn between her love for her brother, her friends' reactions, and worry about herself.

Don't Blame the Music by Caroline Cooney (Pacer Books, 1986). The story of an older sister's return from college with a mental illness.

Only My Mouth Is Smiling (William Morrow & Co., 1982) and its sequel *Crazy Quilt* (Bantam, 1986) by Jocelyn Riley. Thirteen-year-old Merle increasingly hides her feelings from classmates, a new boyfriend, and her grandmother about her mother's bizarre behavior. In the sequel, she and her siblings come to terms with the anger and confusion engendered by their mother's mental illness.

The Keeper by Phyllis Reynolds Naylor (Atheneum, 1986). With his father's paranoia becoming increasingly severe, sixteen-year-old Nick eventually seeks help.

Firsthand Descriptions of Experiences with Mental Illness

A Beautiful Mind: The Life of Mathematical Genius and Nobel Laureate John Nash by Sylvia Nasar (Touchstone, 1998). A well-written account of the brilliant mathematician who developed schizophrenia in his twenties. He received a Nobel Prize for Economics in 1994.

A Brilliant Madness: Living with Manic Depressive Illness by Patty Duke and Gloria Hochman (Bantam Books, 1992). This book intertwines Patty Duke's struggle with bipolar disorder with information about the symptoms, possible causes, and treatments.

Is There No Place on Earth for Me? by Susan Sheehan (Random House, 1983). A searingly realistic account of a woman's experience with mental illness. It includes a good description of historical and political influences on treatments, legal, and funding issues.

On the Edge of Darkness: Conversations About Conquering Depression by Kathy Cronkite (Doubleday, 1994). A series of interviews with well-known people, including Joan Rivers and Mike Wallace, about their personal experiences with depression. Professionals also discuss the illness and its treatments.

The Voices of Robby Wilde by Elizabeth Kytle (Seven Locks Press, 1987). This is an alternately autobiographic/biographic account of Robby's struggle with schizophrenia, which began with hallucinations when he was nine. A very touching and absorbing book.

An Unquiet Mind: A Memoir of Moods and Madness by Kay Redfield Jamison (Knopf, 1995). A powerful, insightful, and eloquent personal account of life with bipolar disorder by a psychologist and authority on mood disorders.

Holiday of Darkness by Norman Ender (Wiley & Sons, 1982). A psychologist's personal journey through his bipolar disorder. Includes a discussion of treatments.

Call Me Anna by Patty Duke and Kenneth Turan (Bantam, 1987). An autobiography of Patty Duke, her struggle with manic depression, and eventual coming to terms with it.

Books for or About Children and Teenagers

Understanding Mental Illness for Teens Who Care About Someone with Mental Illness by Julie Johnson (Lerner Publications, 1989). Written in a language and style teenagers will understand, common misconceptions are dispelled and mental illnesses are described along with suggested family coping strategies.

Children and Adolescents with Mental Illness: A Parent's Guide by Evelyn McElroy (Woodbine House, 1988). Offers a realistic and practical discussion of the problems parents face when dealing with a child who has a mental illness, and suggestions about handling the many decisions to be confronted.

Personal Experiences of Families of People with Mental Illness

The Family Face of Scizophrenia: Practical Counsel from America's Leading Experts by Patricia Backlar (Tarcher/Putnam, 1994). Seven narratives about families with a member who has schizophrenia. Each is followed by advice from professionals about the issues raised.

Families in Pain: Children, Siblings and Parents of the Mentally Ill Speak Out by Phyllis Vine (Pantheon Books, 1982). Interviews with relatives of people with mental illness paint a vivid portrait of the impact of mental illness on all members of the family.

Conquering Schizophrenia by Peter Wyden (Knopf, 1998). The story of the author's son's twenty-five-year battle with schizophrenia. The history of the search for effective treatments is described through the experiences, ups, and downs of the author's son. This accounts ends well with extremely positive results from the use of Zyprexa.

We Heard the Angels of Madness: One Family's Struggle with Manic Depression by Diane and Lisa Berger (William Morrow & Co., 1991). A mother's account of her eighteen-year-old son's return from college and the onset of his manic-depressive illness.

Financial Planning

Planning for the Future: Providing a Meaningful Life for a Child with a Disability After Your Death, Third Edition, edited by L. Mark Russell (American Publishing, 1995). Includes valuable information about government benefits, wills, trusts, estate planning, power of attorney, and more. Especially useful for parents worrying about what will happen to their ill child after they are gone.

Research, Literature, and Books
Written for Professionals

Helping Families Cope with Mental Illness, edited by Harriet Lefley and Mona Wasow (Harwood Academic Publishers, 1994). Family-professional relationships, services for families, training and research, and future directions.

Psychiatric Rehabilitation by William Anthony (Boston University, 1990). An overview of the attitudes, programmatic elements, and strategies of psychosocial rehabilitation.

Schizophrenia: Family Education Methods by Christopher Amenson, Ph.D. (Pacific Clinics Institute, 1998). An overview and manual for working with families of people with a variety of serious mental illnesses.

Family Caregiving in Mental Illness by Harriet Lefley (Sage, 1996). Comprehensive overview of roles families play in caring for relatives with mental illness. Discusses historical perspectives, different family members, and life-cycle issues.

The Role of the Family in Psychiatric Rehabilitation, edited by LeRoy Spaniol, Anthony Zipple, Diane Marsh, and Laurene Finley (Center for Psychiatric Rehabilitation, Boston University, 2000). Intended as a teaching tool for professionals. Provides an organized way to address professionals regarding the needs of family members. Compiled largely from previous publications by the editors.

An Introduction to Psychiatric Rehabilitation, edited by LeRoy Spaniol et al. (International Association of Psychosocial Rehabilitation, 1997). The best articles of twenty years of the *Psychosocial*

Rehabilitation Journal, plus new articles and perspectives by leaders in the field.

Working with Families of the Mentally Ill by Kayla F. Bernheim and Anthony F. Lehman (Norton, 1985). An excellent overview of how to work with families in light of the literature and experience about what families really want and need.

Family Education in Mental Illness by Agnes Hatfield (American Psychiatric Press, 1990). Written by an educator, researcher, and pioneer in the area of working with families, this research-based text focuses on teaching practicing professionals how to work with families of people with mental illness.

Family Therapy in Schizophrenia, edited by William R. McFarlane (Guilford, 1983). Describes several educational and family-therapy approaches to treating schizophrenia. The chapter by I.R.H. Falloon and R. P. Liberman, "Behavioral Family Interventions in the Management of Chronic Schizophrenia," provides research on the effect of family education and family-skills training on the relapse rate of people with schizophrenia.

Schizophrenia and the Family: A Practitioner's Guide to Psychoeducation and Management by C. M. Anderson, D. J. Reiss, and G. E. Hogarty (Guilford, 1986). Describes ways researchers work with families to give support, help them understand the disease, and create a low-stress home environment that minimizes the likelihood of relapse.

Family Care of Schizophrenia by I. Falloon and C. McGill (Guilford, 1987). Presents a review of literature, research, various theories, and techniques for working with and educating families about mental illness.

Addiction, Recovery, and Dual Disorders

Staying Sober: A Guide for Relapse Prevention by Terence Gorski and Merlene Miller (Herald House/Independence Press, 1986). One of the most clear, concise, thorough descriptions of addiction and the process of recovery for those struggling with addiction and for their loved ones.

Wellness Recovery Action Plan (WRAP) by Mary Ellen Copeland (Peach Press, 1997, revised 2000) and *Wellness Recovery Action Plan (WRAP) for Dual Diagnosis* by Mary Ellen Copeland (Peach Press, 2001). Excellent tools for consumers wanting to take charge of their recovery from mental illness or from mental illness and substance abuse. Addressses how to best include family and other support people in the process.

Readings in Dual Diagnosis, edited by Robert E. Drake (International Association of Psychosocial Rehabilitation Services, 1997). This book brings together information from many of the preeminent researchers and clinicians in the challenging field of mental illness and substance abuse.

The Dual Disorders Recovery Book (Hazelden Information and Education Services, 1993). Helps individuals with dual disorders develop a plan for daily living. Personal stories and professional insights create a framework for successful daily living.

The Twelve Steps and Dual Disorders by Tim Hamilton and Pat Samples (Hazelden Educational Materials, 1994). A guide to using the Twelve Steps in recovery from addiction and mental illness.

Co-dependence

Codependent No More, Second Edition by Melody Beattie (Hazelden Information and Education Services, 1997). An excellent description of the syndrome of co-dependency. The problematic effects of excessive and prolonged focus on another individual (such as an ill relative) and how to recover from such patterns.

Hidden Victims: An Eight-Stage Healing Process for Families & Friends of the Mentally Ill, Second Edition by Julie T. Johnson (PEMA, 1994). Filled with vivid personal accounts and case histories, this book focuses on co-dependency and how to be a positive caregiver without losing sight of your own needs.

Deinstitutionalization and Public Policy

Madness in the Streets: How Psychiatry and the Law Abandoned the Mentally Ill by Rael Isaac and Virginia Armat (The Free

Press, 1990). A well-researched description and history of the laws regarding involuntary commitment and deinstitutionalization, and the contribution these have made to so many people with mental illness becoming homeless.

"Administrative Planning in Community Mental Health" by Douglas Polcin (*Community Mental Health Journal,* Vol. 26, pp. 181–192, 1990). A good summary of the history and political forces impacting the community mental system in the United States over the past several decades.

Videos

There is an ever-expanding list of audio and videotapes available. In recent years, researchers, clinicians, public television documentary makers, and fiction film artists have all made contributions to educating the public about mental illness. If you prefer to learn or to help educate others you know through one of these medias, contact your local or national NAMI office for information on how to rent or buy tapes.

Bonnie Tapes: Mental Illness in the Family, The Video, 26 minutes. *My Sister Is Mentally Ill, The Video,* 22 minutes. *Recovering from Mental Illness, The Video,* 27 minutes (The Mental Illness Education Project, Inc., 1997). Each of these three tapes addresses the impact of mental illness through conversations with various family members and with the woman struggling with the illness.

Families Coping with Mental Illness. Comes in both a 22- and 43-minute version (The Mental Illness Education Project, Inc., 1996). Ten people discuss the impact of having a relative with schizophrenia or bipolar disorder. Includes examples of avoidable mistakes, suggestions for family members, how to set limits and maintain a life of your own. While designed to provide support for families, it is also instructive for professionals about the needs of families when mental illness occurs.

Uncertain Journey: Families Coping with Serious Mental Illness, 45 minutes (Duke University Medical Center, 1996). Describes the effects of serious mental illness from the family perspective. Viewers are sensitized to the family experience of serious mental illness through the stories of three families.

Understanding Schizophrenia, Depression, and Addiction, 60 minutes (Adult Science Literacy Project for Mental Health and Addiction, 1995). A tool kit with three 20-minute segments. The focus is on research into physiological and biochemical causes that can lead to destigmatization of these illnesses. The kit includes presentation guides and fact sheets.

Living on the Edge, 55 minutes (The Clinical Research Center for Schizophrenia and Psychiatric Rehabilitation at UCLA, UCLA Psychiatric Research Consultants, Box 2867, Camarillo, CA 93011 (805) 484-5663, *www.psychrehab.com*). About how families cope with mental illness from its onset through the first hospitalization and continuing care.

A Place to Come Back To, 30 minutes (Pathways to Promise— Interfaith Ministries and Prolonged Mental Illness, available from Seraphim Communications, *www.seracomm. com*). Describes mental illness and helps religious congregations learn how to respond to people with mental illness and to develop service projects to help them.

Adult Children of the Mentally Ill, 30 minutes (Dallas NAMI, 1990). An excellent description, by six people who have a parent with mental illness, of the feelings and experiences they go through in learning to cope with the situation.

When the Music Stops . . . The Reality of Serious Mental Illness, 20 minutes (NAMI, 1987). Presents interviews with families and research information about schizophrenia.

Love Story: Living with Someone with Schizophrenia, 42 minutes (1991, available from Wellness Reproductions, 1-800-669-9208). Dr. Frese and his wife describe the knowledge and wisdom they have gained living with the everyday realities of schizophrenia. A hopeful, informative video.

Negative Symptoms in Schizophrenia, 60 minutes (University of Iowa Hospitals and Clinics, 1995). A two-part description of these symptoms and the prognosis for their elimination, by scientist-researcher Nancy Andreasen, M.D., Ph.D.

Full of Sound and Fury: Living with Schizophrenia, 50 minutes (T.V. Ontario, 1985). An extremely poignant and informative portrayal of living with schizophrenia before 1985. Compassionately portrays two people who suffer with schizophrenia and the mother of a man who suicided because of it.

Dark Glasses & Kaleidoscopes: Living with Manic Depression, 33 minutes (National Depressive and Manic-Depressive Association, 1999). Explores the symptoms and treatment of bipolar disorder through honest, emotional testimony of people who live with the illness.

Learning to Live with Bipolar Disorder, 15 minutes (NAMI, 2000). Features five people speaking openly and frankly about living with bipolar disorder and striving for recovery.

Breaking the Dark Horse: A Family Copes with Manic Depression, 33 minutes (Writer's Group Productions, 1994). The person in this documentary struggles with rapid cycling bipolar disorder, yet lives a productive life partially because of a supportive family. Helpful for family members and providers working in the field of mental health.

Depression: Beyond the Blues, 60 minutes ("Good Morning America" ABC series, 1993). Dr. Tim Johnson, with guest experts and people living with the illness including actress Patty Duke, explores myths and facts about depression, focusing on causes, treatment, prognosis, and suicide.

Depression: The Storm Within, 28 minutes (American Psychiatric Association, 1991). Stories of several people, including children, whose lives are altered by depression.

An Integrated Model for the Treatment of People with Co-Occurring Psychiatric and Substance Disorders, 2 hours (available through Mental Illness Education Project, 2000). Lecture by Kenneth Minkoff, M.D., a dynamic speaker and nationally known expert in dual diagnosis. He describes how care for mental illness and substance-use disorders can be integrated despite traditional differences in treatment philosophy. Includes a set of handouts. Geared toward mental-health and substance-abuse professionals.

Informative brochures, booklets, and videos about mental illness can be ordered from some of the organizations listed below. Some also provide information about support groups.

NAMI (formerly called National Alliance for the Mentally Ill)
2107 Wilson Boulevard, Suite 300
Arlington, VA 22201-3042
(703) 524-7600 or (800) 950-6264

National Institute of Mental Health (NIMH) Public Inquiries
6001 Executive Boulevard, Rm. 8184, MSC 9663
Bethesda, MD 20892-9663
(301) 443-4513

Depression and Bipolar Support Alliance (DBSA) (formerly National Depressive and Manic Depressive Association)
730 North Franklin Street, Suite 501
Chicago, IL 60610-7224
(800) 826-3632

Recovery, Inc.
802 N. Dearborn Street
Chicago, IL 60610
(312) 337-5661

American Psychiatric Association
1000 Wilson Boulevard, Suite 1825
Arlington, VA 22209-3901
(800) 368-5777

National Mental Health Association
2001 N. Beauregard Street, 12th Fl.
Alexandria, VA 22311
(703) 684-7722

National Alliance for Research on Schizophrenia and Affective Disorders (NARSAD)
60 Cutter Mill Road, Suite 404
Great Neck, NY 11021
(516) 829-0091

The Mental Illness Education Project, Inc.
P.O. Box 470813
Brookline Village, MA 02447
(617) 562-1111

The Library Media Project
1807 W. Sunnyside, Suite 2A
Chicago, Illinois 60640
(800) 847-3671

**International Association of Psychosocial Rehabilitation
    Services** (IAPRS)
601 N. Hammonds Ferry Road, Suite A
Linthicum, MD 21090
(410) 789-7054

There is an enormous amount of information available on the Internet. Some of the more useful websites are listed here:

NAMI (formerly National Alliance for the Mentally Ill):
    www.nami.org
National Institute of Mental Health: *www.nimh.nih.gov*
National Mental Health Association: *www.nmha.org*
United States Department of Health and Human Services Substance Abuse and Mental Health Services Administration
    (SAMHSA): *www.mentalhealth.org*
American Psychiatric Association: *www.psych.org*
The Schizophrenia Society of Canada: *www.schizophrenia.ca*
National Alliance for Research on Schizophrenia and Depression
    (NARSAD): *www.narsad.org*
Depression and Bipolar Support Alliance (DBSA):
    www.dbsalliance.org
National Mental Health Consumers' Self-Help Clearinghouse:
    www.mhselfhelp.org
Recovery, Inc.: *www.recovery-inc.org*
Mary Ellen Copeland's website: *www.mentalhealth
    recovery.com* or phone (802) 254-2092

Alcoholics Anonymous: *www.alcoholics-anonymous.org*
Alateen and Alanon: *http://www.al-anon.alateen.org*
Narcotics Anonymous:*http://www.na.org*
Dual Recovery Anonymous (DRA): *www.draonline.org*
National Empowerment Center: *www.power2u.org*
Mental Illness Education Project, Inc.: *www.miepvideos.org*
Library Media Project, Video and Electronic Resources: *www.librarymedia.org*
International Association of Psychosocial Rehabilitation Services: *www.iapsrs.org*

Professional Journals

Community Mental Health Journal
Hospital and Community Psychiatry
International Journal of Psychosocial Rehabilitation
Journal of Clinical Psychiatry
Schizophrenia Bulletin
Schizophrenia Research

Index